Version One Is Better Than Version None

21 Secrets to Build Your Strong Version

By

KR Goswami

Dedicated to

My Daughter Miss Hiral Goswami,

Senior Engineer (Software)

Table of Contents

Introduction viii

Chapter 1: Rise Everyday with A purpose.................................1

Chapter 2: Secret of Goal Setting 10

Chapter 3: Things You Do Not Know About Yourself.......................19

Chapter 4: Build Your Strong Personal Brand 25

Chapter 5: Every Hour Counts 36

Chapter 6: Environmental Effect on Human Behavior......................42

Chapter 7: From Novice to Ninja..49

Chapter 8: Become Your Best When Life Gives You Its Worst ..54

Chapter 9: Turn Ideas to Reality 59

Chapter 10: How Not To Talk 70

Chapter 11: Learn Something New Everyday...............................76

Chapter 12: Skills Are Cheap But Passions Are Priceless 83

Chapter 13: The Best Version Of Yourself 87

Chapter 14: Balance Your Pain and Pleasure 92

Chapter 15: Emotional traits transient................................98

Chapter 16: Amount of Sleep 109

Chapter 17: Limited Resources or Unlimited Resourcefulness 113

Chapter 18: Mirror Neurons: Causing Change Within Others. 117

Chapter 19: Connect To Your Inner Self 122

Chapter 20: Adapt to A Changed World 128

Chapter 21: Richness Of Human Life...............................137

Epilogue/Conclusion 144

Bibliography 145

Acknowledgments 146

About the Author...147

Introduction

When I was in Indian Air Force and flying in the chopper, the pilot planned sortie primarily based on the assumptions. Taking off at helipad, landed at the destined place, and gave room for an emergency landing if something went wrong. He covered all the checkpoints before taking off, but he knew that all the identical decisions would be made on the way.

He never tried to forecast for the entire root rather than picking up the current weather report available at the time of take-off, as it was needed to adjust in real-time situations and never stuck. The sit, try and work out every possibility were always available, but the flight plan he took on take-off was always the version one. The project that he ended up executed by the time we landed at our destination was probably Version four or five.

Another example of version one for me while making videos for uploading to YouTube was the biggest challenge when I pushed through the first clip. But I continued with my plans to serve and give to the target audience via narrating a couple of great stories that happened to me. And ultimately, my 21st video was much more attractive than my first video.

In any journey, whether it is a stage presentation, podcast episode, cycling race, or writing book, version one of them was nowhere the robustness of version nine. It was always my first time in every prevailing situation that met the tire with the rugged road, but as long as a Suck Less next time, the newer version was always better than the previous & I could keep on moving till I achieved momentum. If you fall out of speed, then you are dead in the water.

So often, we can be paralyzed by fear. Becoming stuck at the weight of a decision and not wanting to "make a bad decision."

This slowing down of our thought processes is really counterproductive, and it should not be allowed to be your default mindset to set in your business brain. The secret to enabling yourself to make decisions and keep moving is as easy as reciting my favorite saying,

"Version One is better than Version None."

Chapter One: Rise Everyday with A purpose

"Before you eat the elephant, make sure you know what parts you want to eat."

-Todd Stocker

If you have ten tasks in your hands ranging from small to more prominent, you are sometimes confused about which task should be undertaken first and which task at last. Psychologically, we always feel like taking easy tasks first. For example, our teacher asked us to answer easy questions first in the examinations and leave the difficult ones to attempt later. The idea behind picking up small or more manageable questions first is to avoid stressful situations initially so that we can perform better in the later part of the examination. But in a real-time situation, that mindset may not work correctly, especially with tasks involving some long-term projects.

Handle the Bigger Task First

During our primary school projects, we were explained by our teacher with an example of filling a container with certain substances, like stone, sand, wooden logs, water, etc. First, we all loaded the glass container with sand and tried to adjust the rocks in it. But we failed after putting few stones in the container. The teacher then explained the admirable principle of catching up with heavy tasks first. According to the direction, we place more giant rocks first in the container than smaller stones, wooden pieces, then thick sand and thinner sand, and then water. As a result, we accommodate 140% more substances in the container than we had placed the way earlier. In the same way, we can accomplish more significant tasks first and then gradually deal with smaller tasks for more efficient output.

Turn the Pain into Purpose

A task that you are undergoing sometimes makes you feel dull for many reasons; although the job is necessary and sometimes there is no alternative without accomplishing the task. The human mind always tends to adapt two things, it loves happiness or hates pain. But we should also understand that some of the pains are necessary to be happy at later stages. For example, you do not like to go jogging or exercise like stretching or strengthening the body. But we know that chronic pain in the form of exercise helps us be healthy, and we do not easily fall sick later.

In the same way, there are some critical tasks or projects we do not feel like undergoing and therefore procrastinate. List out all of the functions and give an index as per their qualities and quantities. Give priorities to more significant tasks first and then relist in decreasing order. Handle the more essential tasks one by one. Suppose these are the tasks that are to be accomplished in a day; most of the more significant tasks will be finished. You are not much bothered if some of the smaller tasks are leftover at the end of the day.

Salami Slicing

I like the concept of Salami Slicing. It is a series of tiny little actions called clandestinely. It is a combination of little tasks accumulated later as a more significant single task that might not have been possible to perform. It is just like penny-saving considered to be a fraudulent practice of stealing money repeatedly in minimal quantities, usually by taking advantage of rounding to the nearest cent (or other monetary units) in financial transactions. It would be done consistently by rounding down and putting the fractions of a cent into another account. I used to scrutinize my savings bank accounts frequently. Whenever interest was deposited in the account with a predetermined period, the amount was becoming odd. Therefore, I deposited or transferred some money to make it in the round figure to the nearest hundred. This small adding becomes an enormous amount increasingly over a period of time.

IN ONE WAY, when I am writing these words, it is salami writing for my publication, sometimes also referred to this salami slicing. It is a strategy of dividing the results of a single research project into several journals, primarily when aimed at getting more significant recognition of the work. My small paragraphs are forming the part of subheadings, and ultimately, they are my outlines of the book.

Definite Purpose of The Day

You just think when you are coming out of the home and going to market. When nothing is in your head and just going to the nearest mall, it will be just like a football game without a goal post. However, when you want to bring milk and some fruits, you come out of your home with a purpose. You purchase a particular item and return to home. In the same way, when you get up in the morning and do not rise with a specific purpose, your day is wasted. Therefore, it is better to write a list of goals for the next day before you retire to bed. Just like salami-slicing, when everyday purposes are finished, your more prominent and more significant tasks for the week or month are achieved with surprises. Together these accumulations of accomplished tasks become your mission in life.

For the concrete results, all you need to write a significant definite purpose called chief objective. If you commit to some tasks and endure for quite some time, one way, you are constantly feeding your subconscious mind. Your thoughts and purposes are playing the role of stimuli and responses. Carrying out small tasks repeatedly provides your mind a proper thinking process to achieve your chief aim. The repetition of a specific statement has the power to influence your subconscious mind. Your burning desire will also force you to take daily action that moves you towards attaining your goals.

The Great man Bruce Lee had given his chief aim as following,

My Definite Chief Aim:

I, Bruce Lee, will be the first highest paid Oriental superstar in the United States. In return, I will give the most exciting performance and render the best of quality in the capacity of an actor. In Starting 1970, I will achieve world fame, and from then onward till the end of 1980, I will have $10,000,000 in my possession. I will live the way I please and achieve inner harmony and happiness.

-

Bruce Lee
Date: 1969

According to the Ofpad, the school of genius[1], there are following seven steps to make your primary definite purpose,

Step 1 – Determine Your Specific Desire

Determine precisely what you desire, being as specific as possible. You can never have a burning desire for something vague. For example, wanting to be rich is unclear, but wanting to make a million dollars is being specific. Likewise, wanting to lose weight is vague; wanting a 30-inch waistline is being transparent.

Step 2 – Establish the End Date

---

[1] Source: ofpad.com

Establish a date by which you want to acquire or achieve this thing that you desire. It is essential to be realistic. The time period should be long enough for your goal or desire to be achievable but short enough for you to find it worth pursuing.

Step 3 – Determine the Price

Determine what you are willing to give in return for this thing that you desire. You have to pay the price for the object of your desire, and you have to pay it in full before you get it. You never get something for nothing, and the definite chief aim prepares you to pay the price as and when it is necessary. If you want to be a millionaire, you need to create the required value in return for the money. If you're going to get in shape, you have to put in the necessary work and follow a proper diet plan. Regardless of what you desire, there is a price you have to pay for it.

Step 4 – Make an Imperfect Plan

Make a definite plan to help you realize this desire and immediately put this plan into action, whether you are ready or not. Your plan need not be concrete. You just need to start somewhere, so come up with whatever plan you can think of. Note that you need a place to start and a direction to work towards. You don't need a well laid out elaborate plan. Your plan will evolve in your subconscious, and you will think of several different plans at a later date as you start having a burning desire.

Step 5 – Write A Concise Statement

Write the results of the above four steps in a concise statement. It must include what you desire, what you are going to give in return for your object of desire, along with the time limit and the plan with which you intend to acquire this object of your desire. Remember to write down the date when you wrote it down along with your name or signature. This concise statement is your principal definite purpose or definite chief aim.

Step 6 – Reading Your Major Definite Purpose

Read this concise statement twice daily, once after waking up and once before going to sleep. When you read this statement, see and believe that the object of your desire is waiting to be transferred to you as and when you deliver the service/work you have committed to render in return for it in step 3. Reading it aloud is intended to condition your subconscious mind to develop a burning desire by making you constantly think about it.

Step 7 – Changing Your Identity

Repeat the daily reading of your principal definite purpose until you start taking consistent daily action that moves you towards your end goal. Every day, if you are doing something that moves you towards your goal, your definite chief aim has become part of your identity. You can continue to read your primary definite purpose daily if you wish to do that, but I generally revisit my definite chief aimless frequently when I reach this stage. A lot of us get stuck in the planning phase without taking action. You must put your plan into action and progress towards your goal every day through the execution of your plan.

To sum up, I remember Napoleon Hill said, "Whatever the mind can conceive and believe, the mind can achieve." Years of experience of writers from Napoleon Hill to Andrew Carnegie provided the depth of their studies of individuals for the pinnacle of success in their field.

As far as the direction and destination are concerned, I am reminded of my early days of military life when we traveled in choppers. When not calibrated, the navigating instruments were away from our destination and had difficulty reaching the destined place in time. As a result, we had moments of force landing at some of the jungles away from the city.

The aircraft had the specific equipment and technology to travel to virtually any destination. A helicopter had a hull to displace the air and clouds to keep it flying till we reach the destination. The aircraft had an engine with a turbine to produce momentum and lead to directions with a rudder that could direct the aircraft in any specific direction when appropriately used. But the navigational equipment tells the pilot where the plane is and helps guide it along the planned path. What it did not have was the planned path built-in and is provided by the navigator and following the analogy then the pilot of your aircraft. The crew navigating planned the endpoint for the voyage and assisted the pilot with directing the aircraft along the path toward the final destination. If the pilot was performing well, he would begin the journey with a destination port in mind and then start directing us to follow the best path and avoid such things as turmoil and storms that could spell defeat. When the inevitable storm crops up from time to time, the pilot guided us to take necessary steps to weather and the storm but always with the final destination.

The compass showing an un-calibrated needle leads kilometers away from the destination. The same things happen to purpose in life when we do not have a minute direction.

Chapter Two: Secret of Goal Setting

Most of us are wandering in the past, but very few of us think about our life status in the next few years. Yet, our future life depends upon what we do today. When we sail without an exact proper destination, we are tossed away by the existing waves and likely to be wrecked on a stony island. Having clearly defined goals permit you to concentrate your energy on activities that move you ahead in life. If a compass in a steamer has minor variation in reading, the boat may reach miles away from the lighthouse. A combination of the lighthouse and calibrated compass are necessary to get to the right place.

Thomas Alva Edison, the eminent scientist, had a terrific combination of goal and action. He used to call media and press before even starting his new invention. He always declared that he was going for a particular vision. It has excellent psychology behind this idea. You do not postpone or cancel the idea of reaching your goal since people are behind your back as they know your intentions. So sometimes, fear of people will get you to the action. Edison was so focused on his actions that sometimes, he slept in a chair at midnight while working. When he awoke, he started working and finished the assignment.

Fifty years ago, if you told someone we would have mini computers that could access the world's information, flying cars, or artificially intelligent personal assistants and GPRS, they would have told you that you were crazy. But these are the things somebody had written down and put in his action list and achieved after few years.

The Harvard MBA Study on Goal Setting

The 1979 Harvard MBA study[2] on goal setting analyzed the graduating class to determine how many had set goals and had a plan for their attainment. Interestingly enough, the results of1979 Harvard MBA study are identical to the supposed 1953 Yale study.

In the Harvard Business School MBA study on goal setting, the graduating class was asked a single question about their goals in life. The question was this:

Have you set written goals and created a plan for their attainment?

Before graduation, it was determined that:

- 84% of the entire class had set no goals at all

- 13% of the class had set written goals but had no concrete plans

- 3% of the class had both written goals and concrete plans

---

[2] Source: wanderlustworker.com

The result was interesting; 10 years later, the 13% of the class that had set written goals but had not created plans made twice as much money as the 84% of the course that had set no goals. However, the apparent kicker is that the 3% of the class with both written goals and a plan were making ten times as much as the rest of 97% of the course.

Harvard MBA study on goal setting:

#1 — Set a Highly - Specific Goal

The goal needs to be specific. For example, instead of saying you want to be rich, come up with an exact sum of money. As outlandish as it might seem to you today, it's the subconscious mind's focus on that precise number that alters much of your actions on a daily basis. If you don't write it down, it simply means you don't believe enough in the goal.

Pick the number. It can be $100,000, $1 million, $10 million, $100 million or more. The point? Pick the exact number and a precise time till when you'll achieve it. Maybe you'll say $100 million in 5 years from now. Maybe you'll say $100,000 precisely in 12 months from now. No matter what it is, just be specific.

Also, make sure that this is a measurable number. It has to be measurable so that you can track your progress. The more you can follow on a finite level, the more likely you'll be to achieve your goal. That's why it's also essential to be very exact and specific here. For example, you should pick the date down to the very day that you'll achieve this goal.

#2 — Create Strong - Enough Reasons

Reasons come first, and Answers come second. If you have a strong enough reason to achieve a goal, you'll follow through. If you don't, you'll quit. Think about it. In the past, when you wanted something badly enough, didn't you do whatever it took to achieve it?

The point here is to come up with reasons that go beyond the superficial. Those reasons won't work, I can guarantee you that. When the grounds are apparent, when the going gets tough, you'll get going. But when the reasons are deep, and the meanings run to the core of who you are, you'll push through.

What are some examples of strong-enough reasons for wanting to achieve something? Ask yourself the question until your answer equals the question. For example, if you're going to increase your net worth by $1 million by exactly 12 months from now, why do you want it?

Do you want the extra $1 million in net worth for the right reasons? If you say it's because you want to buy a flashy car and a McMansion, you can forget it. If you say you want it for other, deeper meanings, you just might follow through. So let's just say you want it because you want to stop struggling so much in life.

Okay, that's a good start, but that doesn't run deep enough. Why do you want to stop struggling? Maybe it's because you've never really had financial security, and you're looking to achieve that. So, security is good. Why do you want financial security? Maybe it's because you want to take care of and provide for your family.

Security, family, and freedom are some excellent examples of deep-enough reasons. But it would be best if you put some powerful language behind those single-worded reasons. And you have to make sure that you write all of this down. It's great to have deep-enough reasons, but like your goals, you need to be writing it down so it moves from the abstract into reality.

#3 — Develop a Thorough Plan

No matter how outlandish your goal might seem to others, the only person that has to believe in it at first enthusiastically is you. However, regardless of what that goal is, why you want it, you need to create a plan if you're going to follow through. Without a plan, you're dead in the water.

It doesn't mean you need to know every step you took. In the supposed Harvard Business School study, if it were to exist genuinely, I would postulate that 3% that had a plan put some thought into it, but they didn't know every single step along the way. It was a general sense of direction that would have been fleshed out annually, monthly, weekly, and even daily along the way.

Come up with a plan that's thorough enough so that your goals have direction. Don't be left floundering out there. How are you going to achieve those lofty goals? Create a roadmap that will take you from Point A to Point B. Put enough energy and enthusiasm behind this, even if it takes you days or weeks to complete.

Will you start a business? If so, what kind of business? What are some of the steps you need to do along the way to start that business? Legal requirements? Do you need an attorney? An accountant? Website design? Product manufacturing? What will you do? Detail out the steps, no matter what they are, and try to be as thorough as possible.

If you're going to lose weight, buy a new house, or anything else, create the steps you need to follow to see things through. It is an integral part of achieving your dreams, and without it, you might just find yourself giving up before you make any real progress.

#4 — Take Massive Action

Having a plan is excellent. But if you don't do anything to see your plan through, what's the point? It's easy to see now why few people in that supposed Harvard Business School study on goal setting made so much money. So few people set goals the right way and develop a plan and take massive actions to see things through to fruition.

You have to decide what group you're going to fall under and then find the motivation and inspiration daily to follow through. However, to take action, you'll need to do things like stamp out procrastination. Procrastination, as they say, is the silent killer. It's primarily responsible for the 92% of people that don't follow through with their New Year's resolutions.

Also, in order to take action, you need to ensure you avoid time-wasters by effectively managing your time and quitting your bad habits. If your bad habits are holding you back, you'll be hard-pressed to find the time to take massive action daily towards achieving your goals.

We have all of these distractions in life that it's so easy to get sidetracked. From social media to in-person socializing, over-indulgence in television, and everything in between, it's pretty easy to veer off track, but it's crucial to stay on course. Keep yourself motivated and enrich yourself with a daily dose of inspiration is all you need to keep on track.

If your goals are meaningful enough to you, you'll follow through. You'll do what it takes so that you can become like the 3% group in the Harvard Business School study and not like the other 97% group. And to do that, you have to be willing to go the extra mile.

#5 — Manage, Track and Adjust

Daily goal setting and management of your goals are vital as it helps you to achieve milestones along the way to those bigger long-term goals. Daily goals are great also because it allows you to track your results along the way.

For example, if you set the goal of getting out of debt to the tune of $24,000 within 12 months, you can come up with monthly, weekly, and daily plans to achieve just that. So $24,000 of debt paid off in 12 months means $2,000 per month. That might sound like a lot, but not when you look at things on a more finite scale.

$2,000 per month is roughly $66 per day. How can you save or cut out $66 per day in expenses? How can you also earn some side income to make that number more of a reality? Again, if you're committed enough, you'll find a way. But $66 per day sounds much more conceivable than $24,000 of debt, isn't it?

So, track your results by setting daily goals. Then, if you see that something isn't working out the right way, you can adjust your approach. But, similar to a plane that might veer off course due to air traffic congestion, turbulence, or an oncoming storm, you have to make a shift so you can reach your goals. You can't just give up.

The supposed Harvard Business School study teaches us that accomplishing our goals might be difficult. But it's not impossible. As long as we stay focused on our goals and do the required hard work, we'll get there over time. It just won't happen overnight. Don't expect it to happen overnight. But in time, it will happen. It's only a matter of time as long as we don't give up.

What You sow, so you reap

Many of us spend time doing things that do not help us move closer to our goals. Your future life is dependent on the things you do today. You cannot live your dreams in the future if you spend your life today doing average things. If your vision is to fit within the next year, you will not get there if you keep eating junk foods and avoiding regular exercises.

Chapter Three: Things You Do Not Know About Yourself

I will start the topic with a funny incident.

Four of the orthopedic surgeons were returning after a morning walk. A man was passing through and crossed the road with small little jumps with one leg. One of the doctors commented, "I think he has arthritis!" The second doctor said, " No, no, I feel he has plantar fasciitis." The third doctor said, "But I am sure he has spinal lower motor neurons!" Lastly, the fourth doctor said, " I predict that he has Hemiplegia Seizures!"

By the time man came nearer and asked them," Excuse me, can you guide me? Is there any cobbler nearby? I want to get my slippers repaired."

Everybody laughed. The man did not have any of the above orthopedic problems, but he could not walk properly because his slippers were worn out and needed repair.

1. You know yourself better than anybody else. There are four possibilities for self-knowledge.

2. Some of the things you only know about yourself (For example, your bad nightmares)

3. Some of the things you do not know about yourself but people know (For example, your walking style)

4. Some of the things that you know are known to people as well (For example, your education)

5. Some of the things are not known to anybody, neither you nor people (For example, your hidden potential)

You are the best doctor or psychologist for yourself. You know most of your physical comforts, food habits, preference of associates, your strength, and a few of your weaknesses. Some of the things are by birth, and some of them you acquired from the environment. Nevertheless, some of the following things may be useful for self-analysis.

1. You know what you know; you do not know what you do not know

You know many things, and you may be a master in your field, but few things you have not come across you may not be knowing, or you may not have a proper perspective. For instance, I learned how to get good sleep and emphasized exercise, reading, and meditation. But from a recent article, I knew that adequate consumption and absorption of nutrients play a vital part in a good night's sleep. Some of the things that could be better known from positive criticizers of people too. Some of the things you learn better from your mentors.

For instance, I always used my running shoes for cycling, but one of my coaches explained why it was necessary to use them as outsoles play a significant role in better performance and effects.

2. Your perspective may be biased

Psychological researches show that we do not have limited access and accuracy for self-assessment and introspection illusion and run around the bush without proper guidance. As a result, we sometimes do not realize the actions and implementations despite some of the facts. For example, we often talk about charity but ignore the children at nearby footpath starving due to hunger.

3. Your behavior manifests a lot about you

Your behavior is the outcome of your thoughts. When you behave in a particular fashion, your mindset is understood by the people externally. Your facial expressions, gestures, and body language speak many strange things about you. In fact, you expose your inner faces and make them public that you might not consciously note. For example, you may not be aware of your frequently raising your eyebrow, but your friends may notice it and predict what is happening inside your head. It is sometimes difficult to observe ourselves without help, and therefore, we have to rely upon others for such potent facts.

4. Solitude may sometimes help you to know yourself better

A person has more than 50000 thoughts in his mind, and most of the time, he talks with himself. A person can realize many facts when he gains insight into himself deeply and changes his behavior patterns. Mindful meditation helps self-knowledge that can never be compared along with the external help of others. Sometimes we are alone although we are with everybody, and sometimes, we are with everybody although we are alone. Imagination and visualization have potent effects that are generally developed when the person is isolated. Ralph Waldo Emerson has genuinely quoted, "what lies behind us, and what lies before us, are tiny matters compared to what lies within us."

5.   We sometimes overestimate ourselves than what we are.

There is always an actual performance gap between what we aspire to and what we achieve. There may be one of the psychological reasons for the said gap. During a study for judging the size of a coin, it was found among the children that the size of the coin was hyped by the children rearing from lower middle class compared to upper middle class and affluent. We sometimes overestimate our capacity for ourselves, generally termed as a superiority complex.

6.   Tearing off status may result in a setback

When a person fails in a particular attempt, he may feel torn off, leading to distrust, despair, and even suicidal thoughts. Frequent setbacks due to tearing may be deadly for progress and success. It is also a fact that others will value you the way you love yourself. Concerning the married life, it was found that those who have a more positive attitude toward themselves found greater satisfaction in their relationship the more they received praise and recognition from their other half. But those who habitually picked at themselves felt safer in their marriage when their partner reflected their negative image.

7.   Self-deception may stem from the desire to impress others

Self-deception is a process of denying or rationalizing away the relevance, significance, or importance of opposing evidence and logical argument. Self-deception involves convincing oneself of a truth (or lack of truth) not to reveal any self-knowledge of the deception.

Simple instances of self-deception include common occurrences such as the athlete who is self-deceived in believing that his timings are better than his competitors. The wife is self-deceived, considering that her husband is not having an affair. The jealous web designer is self-deceived in believing that her friend's more tremendous professional success is due to ruthless ambition.

8.   You behave more morally when you are insecure

It is generally thought of as a disadvantage. Still, insecurity is not entirely wrong, for example. Sometimes people are told that they are not generous for charity. Yet, they rush towards the donation box and contribute to a particular cause.

9. Think yourself flexibly, and you will have better performance.

If you view your personality as mutable instead of permanent, you are inclined to work on it and improve in any field you are working in. However, a rigid mindset creates a mental trap that makes it challenging to grow. A permanent perspective is always deadly for growth, and you quickly get discouraged by setbacks, and a single obstacle dents your belief in your ability. As a result, you generally tend to become uninterested and give up.

Chapter Four: Build Your Strong Personal Brand

"Be yourself; everyone else is already taken."

- Oscar Wilde

Personal brand impacts your ability to get the right decision at the right place or status where you should be as per your talent and ability. Identify the strengths that make you unique. Think about the traits you can build in each area where you involve yourself. If you are stuck, think about that one area where everyone says you excel.

Self-branding infuses trust and credibility in your knowledge and your abilities. Authentically branding yourself by showing your personality is an excellent way of differentiating yourself from others in your field and developing your brand.

Realize that your brand, like business brands, will change as you grow. The best strategy is to choose a particular area you'd like to focus on and let it evolve over time. But, first, determine what you want to be known for. Your brand is more than a reflection of who you are today; it's a blueprint of where you to go.

Of course, it is not to mention that your brand should be your true self and not something you create. The more natural you are, the easier it is to remain consistent over time. Therefore, being consistent is the most critical element of self-branding.

Personal branding may not be the copycat of somebody. You cannot be the Warren Buffets or Mahatma Gandhi. If you are like precisely either of them, you are not you, but you are someone else. You can derive some of the principles from them, but you cannot exactly copy them. Every individual has a unique personality. There is nobody the same in this world, not even identical twins. The combination of inherited qualities and external learnings from the environment leads to a unique personality. However, the type of associations and quality of reading material plays a vital role in building up the unique personal brand. Several following tips may drastically change the quality of personal branding.

Determine What You Want to Be

Martha Beck[3] shares the four steps you need to visualize the best solution - and then make it happen.

Step 1: Pushback

While visiting China, I heard a story of a wise man there who taught his acolytes by holding a little songbird on his finger. When the bird tried to leave, he'd drop his hand so it couldn't get enough lift to fly away. Lesson: The ability to soar often depends

---

[3] Source: www.oprah.com

upon pushing back against something, you don't want. My feminist friends and I did lots of this; every time we identified things that felt wrong to us in a deeply authentic, visceral way, we were articulating the Pushback.

Since most humans are expert complainers, I'll bet you're feeling some level of Pushback right now. Somewhere in your life, there's a sense of resistance, resentment, discomfort. When babies think this way about pureed liver, they clamp their mouths closed, shake their heads, hurl spoons. Though I doubt you do this at business meetings or parent-teacher conferences, maybe you should. Inwardly, I mean. Outwardly, you can nod and smile the way you always do while noticing the feeling of Pushback.

And when you're ready to start complaining—to your spouse, a cab driver, the pope—don't just bitch and moan. Bitch and moan about precisely the things that bother you. Find the central flaw in the boardroom strategy session. Figure out what exactly about the teacher's condescending attitude makes you want to punch her in the kidneys. The more specific you are about what upsets you and why the clearer you can make your desires.

Step 2: Possibilities

Once you've complained yourself into a wave of high anger, release the energy of finding fault and take up the power of imagination. Holding in your mind the situation that leads to the most vigorous Pushback, begin mentally playing out ways it might change - emphasis on playing. If you feel confined in your tiny office, imagine working in Cinderella's castle, at the beach, on the moon. As Arthur C. Clarke wrote, "The only way of discovering the limits of the possible is to venture a little way past them into the impossible." Each time you feel your Pushback, ride that energy and use it to imagine outrageously fantastic possibilities.

Step 3: Preferences

If you stay loose and relaxed as you're conjuring Possibilities, you'll notice that some of them leave you feeling intrigued, curious, a bit lighter. These are your Preferences. Let them tiptoe into your consciousness. Don't think; just allow. (If you could already think about your Preferences clearly, you'd be creating, not complaining. As T.S. Eliot wrote, "Wait without thought, for you are not ready for thought.") Let yourself form a vague impression, then go for a bit more specificity, as if you're slowly bringing a camera into focus. Allow, and watch.

Step 4: Pinpoints

If you're playful and patient, the Preferences forming in your consciousness will eventually become clear enough to describe in words. You'll begin articulating precisely what bothers you and scenarios you'd prefer to see. Don't jump the gun; hold on a bit longer and get maximum specificity by Pinpointing your desires. Thinking of a solution you'd like to see, ask yourself, what would be even better? After allowing an answer to come into focus, ask, what would be even better than that? Repeat this until you've got an image of a situation so perfect you literally can't imagine a way to top it. This is Pinpoint clarity. Now you're telling the waiter, "Please bring me two free-range eggs boiled for exactly three minutes, seasoned with a dash of sea salt and coarsely ground Tellicherry pepper." That kind of clarity may raise eyebrows, but guess what? It lets everyone and everything around you deliver precisely what you want.

Grow Your Online Presence

When somebody searches your name on Google, it should reflect in the first ten web searches. So to establish your authority figure to increase your brand's reputation. John Rampton[4] has shown four simple methods that will grow your online presence and attract more people you might need them.

1.   Optimize Your Website

At this point, there is no reason why you shouldn't have a website. Surprisingly, however, only 51% of small businesses have a website. That's a significant concern when you have 97% of consumers searching for products and services online. If you haven't done so already, then start getting to work on your website. It doesn't have to be too fancy or complicated. Keep it simple with pages that showcase your work, a bio, contact

---

[4] Source: www.forbes.com

information, testimonials, and a blog where you can share your expertise and unique voice.

Whether you're starting from scratch or updating your existing website, make sure that it is optimized mobile-friendly, loads quickly include a click-to-call button. It also has updated information (work samples, resume, headshots), is easy to keep your eyes on, and optimize URLs easily.

Depending on the nature and size of your business, you may want to take your website a step further and add features like a live chat or create a mobile app.

2.   Choose Your Social Channels Wisely

You've heard time and time again that you need to be active on social media. While engaging and interacting with influencers and customers via social media is one of the most effective ways to grow your online presence, you don't have to be on each and every social media channel. Instead of spreading yourself too thin, focus on one or two primary social channels that you can easily manage and grow.

In most cases, you should focus on the big three; LinkedIn, Facebook, and Twitter. LinkedIn is the preferred choice to network and generates leads, while Twitter is excellent at conversations.

When you find your preferred social network, spend around 20 minutes every day curating content that your customers would enjoy and use tools like Buffer to schedule and manage your accounts. As a rule of thumb, implement that 80/20 rule during your social media campaign - 80% should be shared content created by others, and 20% should be pushing your content.

3.   Go Beyond Blogging

Maintaining a blog not only raises your online presence but also assists with defining your brand's voice and builds trust since you're creating and sharing helpful content. But, you don't want to limit yourself to just blog posts when creating content.

Businesses should be developing multiple forms of content that their customers will either find entertaining or informative Examples include:

Videos that are uploaded onto YouTube or Vimeo.

- Hosting a podcast.
- Creating an infographic.
- Conducting and releasing a case study.
- Publishing an eBook or White Paper.
- Hosting an online course, workshop, webinar.

When you create unique and quality content, it will be passed by industry thought leaders in your industry.

4.   Don't Forget Guest Posts and Email Marketing

Despite all the new tools and techniques out there that promise to help grow your online presence, there are two tried and true methods that shouldn't be neglected; guest posts and email marketing.

Guest blogging, when done for branding purposes and not solely for links, will assist you in earning credibility, help you gain targeted exposure, and increase your website's traffic. For example, let's say that you get a chance to be a guest writer for an established blog or websites like Forbes or Entrepreneur. Those sites have more viewers and authority than your website, which is a win-win for your brand. If that audience enjoys what they've read, then they'll visit your website and hopefully sign-up for your newsletter or follow you on social media.

As for email marketing, McKinsey & Company conducted a study that found "Email remains a significantly more effective way to acquire customers than social media—nearly 40 times that of Facebook and Twitter combined." The main reason is that "91 percent of all US consumers still use email daily." So, when embarking on an email marketing campaign, you should optimize it by segmenting your lists like engaged customers and new subscribers, crafting customized messages, sending your emails at the right time for your audience, and analyzing your data so that you know what tactics have been working and which have not.

Build Network beyond Your Immediate Circle

1. Be a volunteer

Today, most affluent people are contributing their few hours and a handsome amount to raise a cause. It will not help the needy people but also allow you to grow your specific brand with a widespread network.

2. Hoist Events

You must be attending events, sometimes forcefully. Instead of attending your close associates or friend events, it is always better to organize your own event. It will be a prominent act, and attendees will definitely love your role as an eminent host.

3. Gather leads on niche

You can become an expert in a particular niche and start influencing, thereby giving them the value based on principles. Even some companies or entrepreneurs may also have joint ventures and admire your way of organizing such events.

4. Penetrate Through Media

You can successfully represent social media for helping reach fans beyond our natural products niche. With beautiful photos, videos and podcasts, you can quickly reach up to millions of individuals. Provide your audience with great content that they want to look at, and the buzz will spread.

Some of the psychological views

Few psychologists have different views on personal branding. Dale Hartley MBA, Ph.D.Machiavellians[5] has given the following ideas,

These are the reasons that I, as a psychologist, a marketing professor, and as a former business owner and employer, find the concept of "personal brand" to be not only wrong but offensive:

1. Just as companies and organizations should view – and treat – their employees as human beings, not resources or capital, individuals shouldn't facilitate the commoditization of themselves. Yes, you have to market yourself in a competitive economy. You do so by showing past accomplishments and/or your potential to help the organization achieve its goals. In short, what have you done, and what can you do? Ability and achievement are real. Personal branding is puffery (see #2).

2. Is your "personal brand" who you are, really, when you're not working or looking for work? If not, then it's just a false front. You'll never be satisfied and will always feel like an impostor if your reputation is built on false impressions. (I realize that most people behave one way at work, another way with friends, some different way with family, and so on.

---

[5] Source: www.psychologytoday.com

That's not what I'm talking about. I'm talking about act-playing and calling it a "personal brand.")

3. Strong brands are, by definition, limiting. Weak brands are less so. For example, if I ask you to pick me up some Head & Shoulders at the store, you know what I want. But if I ask you to pick up some Suave shampoo, you still don't know which kind of Suave shampoo to buy. If you develop a solid personal brand, you're limiting yourself. If you create a weak personal brand, what's the point, and why bother?

4. Last and probably most important is this: If the idea of developing a personal brand is appealing to you, there might be an underlying problem or weakness you are ignoring. If so, focusing time and energy on developing a personal brand is a distraction from confronting the real issue: Why aren't you content to compete in the job market and the workplace based on merit and who you really are? Do you lack education, experience, self-confidence, or some critical skill? Remedying actual deficiencies is essential. Diverting your attention to personal brand-building while ignoring real issues is a mistake.

However, Human to human touch will spread like wildfire if you have built up the personal brand with principles on true mission and vision.

Chapter Five: Every Hour Counts

"Don't count every hour in the day; make every hour in the day count."

-Unknown

Everybody has 24 hours in their lives. Suppose if one hour is wasted on social media or for some hopeless tasks, can you imagine how many hours are wasted on this earth? There are 7 billion people on the planet. It may amount to a total of 7 billion hours destroyed. But you think if everybody uses their one hour out of 24 hours for productive purpose. There are 7 billion hours of adequate time on earth. This may be achieved because I may not have productive hours at all, and people like me may waste this precious time, but there may be people who may be having more than one hour of adequate time. Some creative people with a growth mindset may have complete 7 to 8 hours of productive time in a day. If we aggregate these hours, there may be more than 7 billion hours of adequate time a day.

Expert Level Performance

K. Anders Ericsson (1947 – June 17, 2020), a Swedish psychologist and Conradi Eminent Scholar and Professor of Psychology at Florida State University, internationally recognized as a researcher in the psychological nature of expertise and human performance.

Ericsson studied expert performance in domains such as medicine, music, chess, and sports, focusing exclusively on extended deliberate practice (e.g., high concentration practice beyond one's comfort zone) as a means of how expert performers acquire their superior performance.

Critically, Ericsson's research program directly complements other research that addresses cognitive ability, personality, interests, and other factors that help researchers understand and predict deliberate practice and expert performance.

He is the originator of studies in which he shared his knowledge that if you want to reach the expert level performance to any narrow field, you have to spend and learn for 10000 hours of practice. After studying professional athletes, world-class musicians, and chess grandmasters, he did the research. He concluded how these high-power competitive folks achieved their ultra-high performing levels in their fields.

Spending 10,000 hours means five years full-time job; anyone can get frustrated. In the year 1972 Summer Olympics in Munich, while winning seven gold medals all in world record time, media people asked Mark Andrew Spitz, an American former competitive swimmer, and nine-time Olympic champion, "So, you must be lucky!" He replied in a very polite manner, " It was not only luck but hard work as well. I worked out 10,000 hours in the swimming pool." It is a necessary calculation here that he must have worked out for 2500 hours every year that is considered 7 to 8 hours work out daily. Ten thousand hours of the practice was emphasized by the author Malcolm Gladwell in his stunning book 'Outliers: The Story of Success' written in 2007, and the book was a best seller for three solid months.

20 Hours of Specific Learning

Best-selling author Josh Kaufman narrowed down this kind of learning in 20 hours. In one of the top 25 most-viewed TED talks, he said that any specific skill you want to know could be mastered with 20 hours of practice. But "If you practice for 45 minutes a day for learning anything, say for instance learning a new language, you can master it in a month. He narrated four following ways to have mastery.

- Deconstruct the skills
- Learn enough to self-correct
- Remove Practice barriers
- Practice at least 20 hours

Lack Of Skills Kills

Any piece of work carried out without skills may be deadly and time-consuming. You can never achieve any type of goal you have aspired without proper skills. Skills are time-saving, and we can devote more time to productive and crucial tasks. There are following few tips thought to be necessary for a better mindset and progress.

1. **Open Mind**

Version One is Better Than Version None

It is said, "Parachute and mind will only work if they are open."
An open mind is a positivity. One should be able to forecast and
explore the possibilities. When half glass of milk is shown,
optimists think half full, but pessimists always think half empty.

2. Lateral Thinking

Explore all ideas which resonate with your passion and niche.
But, first, accept the critical observation of your mentor, who has
a better learning experience. Then, blindly follow the principles
and systems which your mentor has already mastered.

3. Declare Your Research

Your experiments and interpretations are not only worthy for
your records but also stepping stones for your followers. No
records, no access of those nuggets for others. Extracting
methods and modules developed by you may help save
thousands of hours of human resources.

4. Develop Problem Solving Abilities

Problem-solving abilities help treat mental and behavioral
aspects. Unfortunately, problem creators are most hated, but
problem solvers magnetize the people and are liked by people
surrounded.

5. Communicate Better

Any amount of learning skills, research, and inferences are
useless if they are not appropriately communicated. Moreover,

better communication makes the task easy for others to learn things more profoundly.

6. Teach What You Have Learned

You are more than a monk if you learn, implement and teach. The things that you know are useless if you cannot transfer your knowledge to needy people. Moreover, the positive transfer of training or learning facilitates the performance in another context.

Psychology of Productivity

We have ample time in a life span, but there are individual differences concerning productivity. Productivity generally refers to the ability of an individual, team, or organization to work efficiently within the specified time to maximize output. Some people seem to be a natural super contributor or producer; others struggle to become more productive and may look to daily exercises and better habits to help them get things done. An individual's productivity hinges on mental energy and a sense of internal and external motivation. It often emerges naturally from work that they find inherently meaningful or valuable.

Unfortunately, there are countless ways for productivity to be derailed. For example, it takes time for the brain to disengage from one set of tasks and commit to another task, so switching between many tasks at once will slow overall productivity. For example, suppose you are engaged in a coding job in one of the programming modules with deep concentration, but you have been called by your senior to hire you for a moment to some other tasks temporarily. It will take almost 23 minutes to regain your concentration for the last job of coding.

Physical elements boost efficiency and play a vital role in fostering productivity. For instance, exercise, healthy eating, and sufficient sleep produce high productivity results from various aspects like motivation, personality, natural talent, training or education, environment, support from others, time management, and even luck.

Key Take Away

1. Deliberated and dedicated practice for the predetermined period will convert novice to ninja.
2. Document and record every segment of learning skill.

Chapter Six: Environmental Effect on Human Behavior

"The greatest threat to our planet is the belief that someone else will save it."

-Robert Swan

The environment has a significant effect on human behavior. When a baby is born, the behavior patterns make a significant long-lasting effect on the child right from temperature to noise. The child learns the language spoken by his or her parents, and ultimately it becomes the native language. Adults also cannot escape from the predominant effects of the environment. For instance, if you want to shape your body like an athlete or develop your physique like a bodybuilder, it is impossible to live in an inadequate climate where the temperature always remains below 15 to 20 degrees. Even plants do not grow naturally. The different environment produces different kinds of plants, leaves or fruits. For instance, certain fruits like apple and cherry can be grown in colder climates only. There are so many examples of the influences of music on the development of plants. Same watering, but some plants were allowed to grow with music, and some were not. The plants that develop with music grew better than the plants for which music was not allowed. The effects of music are different on man, animal, and plants, which could be seen from the EEG reports, hormone levels, and cell growth.

Repeated Stimuli Is Responsible

Whether it is short or long behavior patterns, there is a typical effect on how living things grow or behave. For example, the rat of the skinner refrained from touching the lever repeatedly after getting an electrical shock from the apparatus. But after that, another rat was taken to the task of connecting the lever that provided food. The responses became automatic after specific repetitions. In the same way, when a human is repeatedly asked to carry out a particular task, his behavior turns to be in clear expectations.

Physiological Aspects

When an experiment was carried out on children, the hungry children overestimated the size of the bread. However, in the same experiment, when children were chosen according to parents' financial status, the children from the lower middle class estimated the size of the coin bigger than the children of the upper-middle class. Therefore, generally, the estimation of the food requirement in the marriage party is not assigned to the hungry person.

In ancient times, man lived in the caves and protected himself from sunlight, thunder, or sunlight. Caves also defended him from wild animals like lions and tigers. Whenever there was a need, he fought with animals and saved himself. Such kinds of external threats have induced stress, but with hiding, running, and fighting, he is externally saved from wild animals. These kinds of fears must have been internally but unconsciously maintained by regulating stress hormones. The immune system of man has become weak during the present time due to subject stress induced in the body due to fear of rejection, fear of illness, fear of taxation, fear of defeat, fear of loss of job, etc. Due to these reasons, man has physically and mentally become weaker despite a lot of facilities.

Love And Belongings

The need for love and belonging from home or society encompasses caring, compassion, empathy, a sense of having a place in the world, being part of a community, feeling accepted, rejected and disapproval, attention, and affection.

Michael Jackson, the American entertainer who spent over four decades in the public eye, employed several doctors for his health ad fitness and had few limbs in spare as he was affluent and wished to live for 150 years.

It is believed that he was physically and psychologically abused by his father, Joe Jackson. The whippings deeply traumatized Jackson and may have led to the onset of further health problems later in his life. Physicians speculated that he had body dysmorphic disorder.

During the 1990s, Jackson had become gradually dependent on prescribed drugs, mainly painkillers and potent sedatives. A high dosage was later linked to second and third-degree burns he had suffered years before.

While preparing for a series of London comeback concerts scheduled to begin in July 2009, Jackson died of acute intoxication after suffering cardiac arrest on June 25, 2009. His physician was convicted of involuntary manslaughter in his death and sentenced to four years in prison.

Self-Esteem

Psychologically speaking, self-esteem is an individual's subjective evaluation of their worth. It is also known as self-worth, self-regard, self-respect, or self-integrity. It encompasses beliefs about oneself. For instance, "I am deprived of facilities," "I am not worthy," etc., or it can be "I am successful," "I can explore possibilities," etc.

An emotional state may be such as triumph and pride or despair or shame. It is a matter of positive or negative evaluations of the self and how we feel about it. Self-esteem is an essential psychological construct because it predicts specific outcomes, such as academic achievement, happiness, or satisfaction in marriage and relationships. It may be an outcome such as abnormal or criminal behavior too. Self-esteem can apply to a specific attribute like "I believe I am a good sportsman and I feel very excited about that") or differently like, "I believe I am a failure, and I feel dejected about myself."

American psychologist Abraham Maslow included self-esteem in his hierarchy of human needs. He described two different forms of "esteem": the need for respect from others in the form of recognition, success, and admiration, and the necessity of self-respect in the form of self-love, self-confidence, skill, and aptitude.

Respect from others was believed to be more fragile and easily lost than inner self-esteem. Yet, according to Maslow, individuals will be driven to seek it and unable to grow and obtain self-actualization without fulfilling self-esteem. Maslow also states that the healthiest expression of self-esteem "is the one which manifests in the respect we deserve for others, more than renown, fame, and flattery." Modern theories of self-esteem explore the reasons humans are motivated to maintain a high regard for themselves.

Emotional Aspect of Environment

Emotion is undeniably the fundamental aspect of the environment. The studies have shown that 38% of what is communicated between people is transmitted through tone of voice compared to the 3% of words. So words are essential, but the intensity becomes more profound with the tone who it is said. So there can be a 180-degree difference of opposite reaction with the addition of subject tone.

I would like to explain it with an example. Assume you are sitting at airport for boarding abroad in aircraft for a pretty important meeting, but suddenly it was announced that the flight is late for a couple of hours due to bad weather. You may get annoyed, rush to the announcer and break the window as it was very much necessary to reach in time for the meeting; otherwise, there might be a heavy financial loss. It might be most likely an upsetting experience and might provoke anger and frustration. But when it was declared, you thought for a while that lousy weather might invite an air crash, and you might be a victim of an accident. Your emotion is regulated through your ability to respond, and you manage your emotional response.

In psychology, there is an exciting term call defense mechanism. When something goes wrong against your will, you think differently and decide and be satisfied for a worthy cause of happening, just like the jackal's "Grapes are sour!" as the grapes hang at a very high position.

Self-actualization

Self is the answer to who we are, how we define, categorize, what do we think about ourselves, and why we believe in that way. Self is a system consisting of eighty self-related phenomena due to three aspects: representing, effecting, and changing. Self is also interconnected in social, psychological, neural, and molecular levels of mechanisms. Self-discovery or self-image are constituted through the experience of self-awareness or self-consciousness or may be deteriorated as self-deception or delusion.

From the environmental stance, the identities of people exist before birth and continue after death. They are in the minds and memories of people even beyond physical existence. The impact remains through social interactions and behaviors they have constructed out of their multiple identities. Some great thinkers have impressed us for better lives and inspired us even though they are not present, and the effect continues even when they have left this planet. So the environmental impacts internalize even after decades.

Self-actualization is, in fact, an subjective experience. Maslow described self-actualization as striving for one's reaching and fulfilling own potential. Thus, the psychological profile of self-actualized people consists of two dimensions as openness to experience (being aware of one's emotions, having insight, empathy, and healthy interpersonal relations), and reference to self (being responsible for oneself, having a well-developed ethical understanding, and self-esteem, expressing oneself cognitively and emotionally and not being too much sensitive to other people's ideas, influences, and criticisms).

These ways show a feeling of trust with an open attitude, choosing development instead of fear and doubt, listening to one's sound inner voices, being honest to oneself, taking necessary steps for being satisfied, not only focusing on ultimate goals. Also, discovering the process of self-actualization, living peak experiences, exploring one's psyche, and having the courage to see and give up defense mechanisms. Thus, in these ways, people can enhance their well-being.

Chapter Seven: From Novice to Ninja

"A breakthrough in machine learning would be worth ten Microsofts."

-Bill Gates

The user interface is where human and computer systems interact with simultaneous use of input devices and software.

Command User Interface

In the old days, when windows were introduced, we were familiar with Command User Interface. We did not like but forcefully remembered specific commands, but we had exciting moments while executing the set of commands. The predetermined results on the command prompt were surprisingly astonishing as it was giving results just like that of a calculator. Only boring keyboard as mouse, joystick or any other modern pointing devices did not exist. Command Line Program that accepted text input and was sufficient to execute operating system functions. In the 1960s, using only computer terminals was the only way to interact with computers. In the 1970s and 1980s, command line input was generally used by Unix systems and PC systems like MS-DOS and Apple DOS.

Graphical User Interface

With the launching of window (3.1), the graphical user interface was in command; however, it was slow, but as far as psychological results were concerned, the visual representation was much more palpable as the subconscious mind always understands the language of pictures and images. CUI is not easily changeable but has high speed and precision. Human has evolved over comforts and therefore always liked and adopted changes that pleased the mind. GUI requires high memory, but usage is easy and highly flexible.

Multimedia User Interface

The interface presented a window to the user for controlling storage and retrieval, inserting objects in the document and specifying the exact point of insertion, and defining index marks for combining different multimedia streams and the rules for playing them back. If you are a fan of music, you must have used tape recorders before a few decades back that were not sequential, and we could not jump randomly for desired songs, but with digitization, we could reach and listen to preferred songs within seconds. It was a great relief for music lovers who had to rewind many songs for minutes to get a particular song in audio and video cassettes. A user interface for multimedia centers advantageously utilizes hand-held inertial-sensing user input devices to select channels and quickly navigate the dense menus of options. Extensive use of the high resolution and bandwidth of such user input devices is combined with strategies to avoid unintentional inputs and with lush and intuitive interactive graphical displays.

HDMI (High-Definition Multimedia Interface) is a proprietary audio/video interface for transmitting uncompressed video data and compressed or uncompressed digital audio data from an HDMI-compliant source device, such as a display controller, to a compatible computer monitor, video projector, digital television, or digital audio device.

With the latest version of iTunes, we are more excited to have musical and other stuff combined in one place. iTunes is a media player, media library, Internet radio broadcaster, mobile device management utility, and the client app for iTunes Store, developed by Apple Inc. It is used to purchase, play, download, and organize digital multimedia on personal computers running the macOS and Windows operating systems and can be used to rip songs from CDs and play content using dynamic, smart playlists. In addition, options for sound optimizations exist and ways to wirelessly share the iTunes library.

Application Programming Interface

Application Programming Interface is a software intermediary that allows two applications to talk to each other. Each time you use an app like Facebook, send an instant message or check the weather on your phone. For instance, you are sitting in a modern restaurant and ordering from your devices. The specific device software is connected with the modular restaurant kitchen; food is served on your table with the help of a waiter or robot. Another example is for the flight booked for your staycation. You fetched the data through an application connected to tourist bus or airline software with predetermined data like date, time, location, etc. With intelligent integration, the data is passed to various other applications, like payment gateways, including email automation sequences that give you instant information and reminders on your android or desktop.

Software as a service (Saas)

It is not outdated to talk about 'Software as a service,' a software licensing and delivery model in which software is permitted on a subscription basis and centrally hosted. It is sometimes referred to as "on-demand software" and was formerly referred to as "software plus services" by Microsoft. SaaS applications are also known as on-demand software and Web-based/Web-hosted software. SaaS is considered as a part of cloud computing and infrastructure as a service (IaaS).

Enterprise resource planning (ERP) systems are the backbone of many organizations, helping them manage their accounting, procurement processes, projects, and more throughout the enterprise. Unfortunately, for many IT departments, ERP systems have often meant large, costly, and time-consuming deployments that might require significant hardware or infrastructure investments. The advent of cloud computing and software-as-a-service (SaaS) deployments are at the forefront of a change in the way businesses think about ERP. Moving ERP to the cloud allows businesses to simplify their technology requirements and see a faster return on their investment.

Cloud ERP solutions are mature offerings that have all the same features and functionality as their on-premises counterparts. In addition, the cloud deployment model easily enables the integration of other key technologies, such as mobility, decision support systems, and collaboration and social systems. As a result, cloud services are growing in popularity among leading businesses that want applications with modern functionality but without the overhead of IT infrastructure, maintenance, and upgrades. To ensure the success of your SaaS ERP system, you can leverage integrated suites and cloud platforms with industry-leading high performance and scalability, unparalleled reliability, and improved security.

The above words emitted from the mind when I was using AJAX (Asynchronous JavaScript and XML)

I have to crack a joke finally.

Rewire your brain and integrate API into the outer world!

Chapter Eight: Become Your Best When Life Gives You Its Worst

"Cats are marvelous creatures - they either adapt to circumstances or decide to make circumstances adapt to them. Either way - they win."

-Will Advise

The intensity of wind during a storm cannot harm the more vigorous trees because the more robust trees have their roots stronger. However, some of the fragile trees may fall and be destroyed as their roots are not strong. In the same manner, no life situation can harm you if you are stronger within. So your thought process should be very much solid and positive so that no external storm of the environment can do any to harm you.

The environment is an opportunity

It depends upon you how do you take it. For example, some people may start complaining that circumstances were not favoring. Still, some people may be swimming against the current and say that I became stronger because the environment was not friendly.

Albert Einstein always said, "It's not that I'm so smart, it's just that I stay with problems longer." So you have to be consistent with yourself how you define yourself.

Version One is Better Than Version None

Tony Robbins once said," One of the most incredible days in human beings' life on the journey of emotional maturity is the day that we realize that life is not a comfort-centric experience but a growth-centric experience."

Power Of Acceptance

If you are complaining about something that has already happened, you are wasting your time. Accept the zero-tolerance policy on your own thinking for any thought that started with "if only" or "what if" why because you can not go back and change anything. What is in your control is your next move to deal with what has happened.

When Thomas Alva Edition saw his factory burning with ashes and thought nothing can be controlled now, he asked his son, "Call your mom; she must not have seen such a huge fire in her life!" When one of his friends came and passed his condolences, he said, "My all mistakes burned, let me start with new ones!"

Millions of dollars were lost, but he never lost his emotion because he had the power of acceptance. Napoleon Hill said, "Within every adversity is the seed to an equal or greater benefit."

Contrast Frames

The contrast effect is a magnification or diminishment of perception due to previous exposure to lesser or greater quality but of the same base characteristics. The term can be learned more clearly with the following two contrast examples.

A) Negative Frame Effect

When my father gave me the mango in my early childhood, I felt pretty well, but after half an hour when my younger brother arrived, my father gave him two mangoes. Although he was my real brother to whom I loved very much, I wouldn't say I liked the way my father acted. Later on, during my psychology practice, I learned that if I have to give a pencil to my son, I will make sure I will give it to my daughter while a partial piece is left with her.

B) Positive Frame Effect

During one of the online digital course webinars, the presenter showed joining fees as $100. The figure was burning in my mind, but later on, when he reduced it to $60 as a particular case for the next 15 minutes, that was cheaper than the first offer. It was a part of sales technique in which the first offer was shown quite expensive than the later that seemed inexpensive compared to the first one. People adapt to change their minds by changing the context in which they see an event or the meaning they give to it.

Man's search for Meaning by Viktor Frankl

During the early days of my training in the Air Force, I had many adjustment problems in my barrack of training camp. We had to put off lights before 10 pm, get up at 5 am for a healthy run, get ready for the parade at 7 am. Learning about fighters and other aircraft from 10 am to 4 pm. Then, we had to again get ready at 5 pm for physical training and workouts. I thought of leaving the training, especially when there was an intension scarcity of water to make us stronger for more challenging times. There was nobody to help me in those days, and finally, I sought my elder brother, a sports teacher, in high school. I can never forget my brother, who left for heavenly abode at the age of 37 years after presenting me a book "Man's Search for Meaning by Viktor Frankl," a memoir of Frankl's imprisonment in concentration camps during World War II. The book had a brief description of the principles of logotherapy, a school of psychotherapy that he founded.

Frankl and his family were imprisoned in concentration camps during the war. Frankl was held in several camps before he was liberated from the last in 1945. During his time in the camps, Frankl witnessed the extreme cruelty of camp guards and the prisoners who were given special status, also known as Capos. He also witnessed the brutality of the prisoners to each other as they underwent the three stages of reaction to their imprisonment. These stages are denial, acceptance, and adjustment after their release.

Frankl discovered that although the prisoners seemed utterly powerless, they had the freedom to choose their reactions to their circumstances. Those prisoners who were most resilient were those who had something to live for!

I never had any complaint of circumstances till now after reading this powerful book.

Key Take Away

1. In any prevailing circumstances, there are two choices. You can continue to be cruel to yourself, or you can be kind to yourself.

2. There are many things you cannot control, but how about the things that you can handle? Take action.

Chapter Nine: Turn Ideas to Reality

"The day before something is a breakthrough; it's a crazy idea."

-Peter Diamandis

Ideas are like a butterfly. They fly away within no time. Therefore, it is advised to keep a pencil or diary/ notepad in the pocket so that your essential thoughts in the form of an idea are not lost. Great ideas always exist, but they are lost due to procrastination. We lose the advantage of a good idea often due to delay in execution or implementation. Successful execution takes consistent, disciplined steps, deep commitment, alignment in direction, and collaboration.

So often we say to our friends or fellow workers, "It is a fantastic idea!", but generally it remains an idea only. The spontaneous idea may be converted into reality if it is immediately processed or sufficient work is done on that very idea; otherwise, it remains dormant. Thus, the idea may be lost forever.

Transforming an idea into a reality is never easy because it demands discipline of actions and organized steps to carry out a particular task. In fact, it is challenging because it is as tricky as nurturing a plant. Generally speaking, when you have a good idea, others are not interested unless they have some benefits. For example, you have imagined the fruits of a tree while sowing the seeds, but others do not perceive it.

Message To Mission

The message of your idea may be converted in mission and result in a moment if the purpose of the concept is strong enough. You should be able to influence the people and convince them regarding the benefits of outcomes or the final result.

Great ideas might be generated in the mind while you are walking, cycling, or practicing meditation. They can also be generated while you are watching television or doing some house chores. When you are silently listening to a podcast or good audio, you may get good ideas. Whatever may be the media, the idea generated should immediately be noted.

Every Trivial Idea Has Value

No idea should be considered minor. Innovative thinking is not required for idea generation. The idea may come from a business person or labor. A fourth-class employee gave the great idea of one day cricket. Laborious five-day cricket has now been converted to T20 via One-Day International. Business of huge amount has never been possible if the clue would not have been converted to reality or if it would have been thought that the trivial idea of a fourth-class employee does not matter.

American entrepreneur, animator, writer, voice actor, and film producer Walter Elias Disney would have never been a pioneer of the American animation industry. The idea would not have been generated after watching a rat playing or eating a piece of bread raising on two legs. Nevertheless, his introduction and several developments in the production of cartoons as a film producer could not have held the record for most Academy Awards earned by an individual, having won 22 Oscars from 59 nominations.

One of the most influential physicists and scientists of all time, Isaac Newton, gave gravitational reality from an apocryphal story about an apple falling on his head. If he had annoyed and thrown the apple in an angry mood as it fell in his head, we would have been deprived of the theory of gravity.

Individual Vs. Organization

In organizations, when employees work, they have a stereotype of jobs. They finished specific tasks allotted to them, and they pack up when time is over. They are not bothered by the organization because the broad idea of innovation is not implied, and training and learning are not designed for individual growth. 'Build the men, and they will build the organization' approach should be emphasized. However, if the employees are involved in a particular type of decision-making role, some ideas are generated in their minds and may be helpful in the organization's growth.

A great contributor Glenn Llopis has given the following 12 things that convert ideas into reality.

1.   Believe in Yourself

You can't take action until you believe in yourself enough to handle the consequences of your decisions. Any time you assume the responsibility to give something that had not existed before an opportunity to become a reality – you become accountable for your actions.

Accountability requires believing in yourself enough to be 100% dedicated to getting the work done. Most people fail to take an idea to fruition because the unexpected challenges become more than they think they can handle, and thus they no longer want to be accountable. They lose the belief in themselves to see things through all the way to the end.

2. Create Your Own Personal Board of Advisors

Learn from those who have done it before. Don't ever think you have all of the answers just because it's your idea. Ideation is distinctly different than execution.

Allow your personal board of advisors to guide you with wisdom born from their failures and subsequent successes. I talked to a couple of fellow entrepreneurs about this, and they offered some of their learning.

Rich Melcombe, President & CEO of Richmel Media & Productions, says that: "If you want to be a successful entrepreneur, listen to everyone because you never know when you will hear a good idea. Advice from stakeholders is usually more meaningful but not necessarily right. Few people will have enough context to understand what you're trying to do fully. So instead, synthesize their comments, so they make sense to you, understand the thinking behind any negative comments, and then make the decision on your own."

Brad Lea, Founder & CEO of Lightspeed VT, adds: "Although it is valuable to have a personal board of advisors, be careful not to let them deter you from your vision. Steve Jobs' board said he was "crazy" to enter into the cell phone space because it was saturated and it would not be worth the long and laborious effort."

In the end, carefully evaluate any input you get – but proceed with your own gut instinct.

3. Embrace Risk as Your Best Friend

Risk becomes your best friend when you give birth to an idea. If you can accept this fact, you will approach the process with a lens that keeps your dreams and ambitions in perspective and on track. When things don't go as planned along the way, stay focused on the mission at hand and do not allow disruption to set you backward. Risk is average, and steps #1 and #2 will keep you looking forward.

You often hear that "working hard" is imperative to convert ideas into reality. But in fact, it is the most fundamental commitment one must make to assume any form of risk management. As such, you must find a way to make this level of commitment if you want to continue on the journey.

4. Be Extremely Patient

Compromise is a choice, not a sacrifice. Don't put too much pressure on yourself. Take the time to appreciate the journey and understand how things work. Most people are too anxious to get their desired results and thus start to make bad decisions as they go.

One thing is sure: the journey will be filled with unexpected outcomes that you may not be prepared to deal with. Don't let this get you down, but keep your head up and respect the process and where it takes you. You will learn a lot about your threshold of risk and ability. Equally, you will realize that many doubters are ready to stand in your way and may attempt to bring you down; this is when the ride gets uncomfortable. Constantly reevaluate those with whom you are sharing the journey (i.e., your inner circle).

5. Learn How to Sell Your Vision

Converting your idea to reality requires you to help others understand your vision. Selling vision is much like selling change. Clearly define your value proposition and how it can generate revenue. Selling lofty ideas without understanding how they will achieve financial results will never get you the right audience. The bottom line is what gets everyone's attention (you can see this played out every week on the TV show "Shark Tank").

Simplicity is the key to selling the vision for your idea. Making it easy for someone on the "outside" to understand what you are trying to accomplish will create engagement and increase your probability of expanding buy-in for your idea. This skill comes into play when selling to possible investors. Learn how to sell your vision sooner than later. Please don't wait, as it takes time to piece together and refine your message.

6. Connect the Dots Along the Way

Everything is connected to something else. Learn how to spot the paths of connectivity along the journey. What may be your "core idea" today can mature into something more prominent as you connect other tenets that naturally associate with your idea along the way.

For example, I launched a food business in 1997 called Luna Rossa Corporation. I started with a product line of specialty vegetables anchored by my flagship product of marinated artichoke hearts. The idea was to market gourmet / higher-quality Luna Rossa branded products inside warehouse retailer Costco – which we successfully accomplished. Over time, this core idea led to gourmet line extensions that included pasta sauces, salad dressings, etc. We sold products to over 6000 retail stores throughout North America, eventually creating new brands and entering into licensing arrangements.

Never stop connecting the dots!

7. Be Passionate With Your Pursuit

The pursuit of excellence requires you to unleash your passion. When you put your love into everything you do, it gives you the power to become a potent pioneer. You will blaze paths few would go down and see them all the way through to the end. Your passionate pursuit of converting your idea into a reality will open new doors to endless possibilities.

Your ability to remain passionate about what you stand for is the ultimate enabler for the success of your idea.

8. Be Purposeful

Your intentions for your idea must have purpose and meaning. If not, your probability of quitting along the way will increase. It will also increase the likelihood of you "psyching yourself out with unnecessary excuses."

Rich Melcombe adds: "Entrepreneurs must have passion and believe in what they are doing, or they are destined to fail. You need to commit to yourself and have a fiduciary responsibility to anyone who supports your idea or concept. Your purpose is to execute the idea and make others believe too."

Purpose fuels your passion and makes your journey less lonely. Perhaps this explains why family-controlled firms outperform their public peers by 6% on company market value. Today, one-third of all companies in the S&P 500 index are run by families.

9. Focus on Building Momentum

Carefully identify all of your resources and build upon them via relationships, networking, and sharing of resources to expand the opportunity for your ideas. Building momentum is critically essential to convert your vision into a reality.

Stay focused, stick to your plan, eliminate distractions, and neutralize the noise. Remember to manage your time wisely and never get overly excited about new opportunities that stem from your original idea. Step back, don't commit too quickly, and understand how the dots connect.

Building momentum has a lot to do with timing and the management and deployment of resources. Every resource counts. Know when and when not to use them, so their value is optimally utilized at the right place and time.

10. Always Make the Idea Better

Never grow complacent. You can continually expand upon your idea and make it better. When you begin to see how the dots connect, challenge yourself and your board of advisors to make your pictures even better.

This is what Steve Jobs did with Apple, Pixar Animation, and Apple again. Continuous improvements were part of his legacy. He never stopped thinking of ways to make his ideas better. The Japanese even have a name for it: Kaizen.

11. Make Work/Life Balance a Priority

No matter how smart, passionate, or focused you work, we are all susceptible to burnout without balance. Mind, body, and soul must be properly aligned. So take the time to make work/life balance a priority. It will give you greater clarity of thought and help you keep things in perspective.

Successfully converting an idea into a reality is a marathon, not a sprint. Pace yourself so that you can reflect upon the mission at hand. Always be aware of what you are attempting to accomplish. Don't overwhelm your mind; give yourself some breathing room and allow your creativity to expand.

12. Build a Legacy Around Your Idea

Let's say you made the commitment to assume the responsibilities associated with the first 11 steps and have already been successful. Your original idea was born, and its impact has now morphed into multiple areas that you would have never thought possible at the beginning.

You have "earned your serendipity," and the opportunities you have created for yourself and others have been influential. The success of your idea is now confirmed; it has become something more significant, and it is up to you to make sure its legacy remains sustainable.

Once you give your idea its life, it is your responsibility that its impact stays alive forever.

> **Key Take Away**
>
> 1. "An idea that is not dangerous is unworthy of being called an idea at all." – Oscar Wilde
>
> 2. "Ideas are easy. It's the execution of ideas that really separates the sheep from the goats." – Sue Grafton

Chapter Ten: How Not To Talk

"Be who you are and say what you feel because those who mind don't matter, and those who matter don't mind."

-Bernard M. Baruch

Humans roughly talk about 60-70% with others. Out of all time, they talk with themselves for the rest of the time. Whether positive or negative, they talk profoundly. You must have seen some individuals who are talking even when they are alone. They derive pleasure while speaking and may sometimes be sad also. The feeling of talking is just like that of food, sex, or other materialist needs. If we know how the brain works and reacts, we can control such talking desirably.

Mesolimbic Dopamine System

Once a person is talking with oneself, he is associated with the mesolimbic dopamine system. The subject system is the roadmap of dopamine traveling from one place to other in the brain. Just like the chocolate of a child, dopamine is responsible for pleasure and reward. The whole internal system of the specific area of the brain is activated by linking to the limbic system. The mesolimbic dopamine system is associated with the functions of movement, preservation, and compulsion.

There are five types of dopamine receptors in our brain. These receptors play a vital role in the brain processes of cognition, motivation, memory, and learning. Here neurons also play a significant role in the synthesizing of dopamine.

Behavior Recognition

Once we know the internal structure or pathways of dopamine and how it travels to other parts, it will be easy for us to control our talking. While talking to others or talking to yourself, you can recognize the undesirable words. You can give little punishment to yourself like pinching to a particular place in the body or closing your eye for some time, or uttering some good gossips. Your good friend may be helpful when you are in conversation and confront such words.

When you are listening to somebody, you generally feel that it is your story. Put the legs in the shoes of the person who is narrating the story. The person is sharing the story with his perspective and observe it in the third person only.

Be vigilant and do not allow yourself to focus on yourself about the narration. For example, when your friend talks about horse riding, do not try to shift the focus to cycling because it is your hobby. Instead, let his preference be confined to him only. Instead of pointing him out your ways, prefer to say, "That is awesome!"

When you are listening with concentration, your full attention is with him, and there are fewer chances of talking to yourself, all most negligible. For example, suppose a friend asks about the readings and says, "What type of books do you prefer to read?" You can tell, " I generally read self-help books and positive mental attitude books." And then you can make him the goalkeeper by saying, "Have you read any self-help book?"

It is always good to be a good listener, but you may not be constructive in your conversation. So it is always better to note down some points and express your opinion later on. It will encourage you to focus on what you want to say according to your point of view.

Your Approach to Conversation Matters

If you may have a good vocabulary, but you may not be a good orator. When your friend is talking, and you are cutting his talk in between because you know the matter better is a bad manner. Let him talk when it is his turn. Allow your friend equal time to talk about himself, giving him your full attention.

You may not always be correct. But, concentrate on what he says and try to learn and grow because what you know you know, but what you do not know, you do not know. Sometimes we stick to our plan and ignore the opinion of our counterparts. The conversation should be like sportsman spirit rather than the interactions against each other.

Prioritize what you can learn. For example, when you are ordering fruit juice, you can say, "I like pineapple because I read vitamin C is there in an adequate proportion." Instead of saying, "you can also take." Prefer to say, "what do you like?" and let your counterpart respond. What he or she prefers matters the most.

Always opine considering your point of view, which may or may not be the other's view. Consider the opinions of others and think for the next level of learning.

Use Specific Conversation techniques

When you have crafted a good subtitle of your book, always give credit that I could have such an excellent book cover only with my friend's guidance. Self-certification is generally considered an aberrant manner. Instead, always illuminate people, for instance, "Your idea of growing more trees is wonderful because ozone layer and oxygen are a matter of concern."

Listening is fantastic art, and therefore listen carefully and try to talk when your counterpart puts the ball in your court. But, again, your body language, like nodding, smiling, raising eyebrows, etc., are essential gestures as they show that you are pretty sincerely engaged in the talk.

Instead of telling 'yes' and 'no,' ask helpful questions. If your friend says, "I like blue color." You can prefer, "Why do you like blue?" instead of simply saying, "yes."

Always validate the statement told by your friend. For example, you can say, "It is one of the most insightful thoughts of yours I have come across!"

There are some vital tips that you can also remember while speaking to a friend or across the audience.

1. Treat Throat Like Piano

Your throat is like a beautiful musical instrument. Others like the sweet voice of the device. In the same way, you can make your voice sweeter through specific practices. Being an artist of All India Radio in singing, I had been undergoing rehearsals to condition the vocal chord to have a sound vibration at definite intensity. Moreover, practicing high and low pitch may add laurels to your speech.

2. Diaphragm Secret

Another critical aspect is the fitness of your lungs and diaphragm in your stomach. Breathing in and breathing out at a specified rate is essential. Your continuous faster breathing may not energize you to talk or address adequately. Some of the breathing techniques, along with yoga and meditation, may add smell to gold.

3. Respiration Is Inspiration

Breath is life. The moment you took birth to the time you will be here, the only process that is with you all the time is breathing. The moment breathing stops, your soul will leave your body. That's why all spiritual teachers remind you to pay attention to the breath.

Version One is Better Than Version None

When you breathe in, feel the love of others, and when you breathe out, feel that you distribute love. Your air inside and the air outside is the love you give and take. Your inhaling and exhaling is the language of the soul.

You desire to live in love, joy, happiness, and prosperity. So inhale all that you like and exhale everything the way people love it. It is the simplest way to transform your life.

Key Take Away

1. "Be careful when you talk to yourself and others."

2. "Always know when you have to shut the mouth."

Chapter Eleven: Learn Something New Everyday

"Live as if you were to die tomorrow. Learn as if you were to live forever."

-Mahatma Gandhi

Most of us have a couple of areas in our life that drive and strive to know well. The primary thing about our job and a hobby or both. Sometimes we know what we know, but we do not know what we do not know. It is therefore advisable to learn something about everything and everything about something. If you do not realize, you perish. If you learn new things, you can teach new things. If you do not learn new things, how long you can teach old things repeatedly. Can you remove darkness with darkness? It is the ray of light that expels darkness. Hate somebody continuously, and you will be hated forever. It is the love that can finish your hates.

The prettiest thing about learning is that nobody can take it away from you. It is stored in your brain, and it is your private property forever. Think how painful it could be to have a 10% wealth tax for what you possess in your brain? In fact, we are blessed to learn anything anywhere, and there is no limit on that. So, you can learn as much as you can.

Do Not Be Afraid to Be Wrong

You may always commit some mistake when you learn new things. In fact, go and commit some mistakes to remember things more deeply and understand better. For example, while coding for your program in my module, I faced more than a dozen of errors when compiled before execution. But it was always version one. Several attempts were eliminated with several attempts, and I jumped with joy when the program was successfully executed. The same thing happened in my job, in sports, swimming, cycling, running at cross country, and running a marathon.

You Can Learn at Any age

Generally, it is believed that learning is possible at school or college days only. But it is a myth. It is also commonly thought that there is no time later on in life to learn things. You can learn anything at any time. Some people laughed in my office when I was learning and applying typing techniques with speed later. But it is the outcome of the same learning that I can present a book every month to the world. One of my friends burst into laughing when recently, after my 60, I took a course on Photoshop even I had uploaded more than one hundred videos on my YouTube channel. It is never too late to learn anything, and no subject is too outdated to learn unless and until it does not lead to your ultimate goal. I had learned to swim at the age of 16 years, but my relatives surprised me when I learn SCUBA diving in the deep water of sea at the age of 58.

Wide Range of Subjects

It will have been a situation with mercy if you are restricted by some authority or a law across the country that if anybody learns more than six things, it will be a punishable offense. So to narrow down your learning to the area of specialization day by day and week by week. It will be exaggerated, but I can learn every hour of the day if you want precisely to get legendary in your field. Psychologically speaking, the mind is not always ready to accept or adapt the changes quickly and frequently to the new situation. Still, you got to make a habit, and ultimately a habit will form you. Once you have succeeded, especially in unfamiliar situations, it will just feed as innovation to hundreds of individuals, thereby thinking creatively and providing examples to follow your pathway. It will impress everybody around you and deepen your own character and make you more confident. So, make your life worth living by learning new things.

Barriers To Learn New Things

Everybody wants to learn things, but everybody can not because there are internal and external factors responsible for hindrances.

A) Internal Factors

1. Mental or Physical State

You are less interested in violence happening around your city than the pain you face in one of your teeth. My friend was not interested in learning gaming skills as his grandmother was seriously ill.

2. Fear of Failure

One of my close relatives did not learn to drive throughout his life because he thought he might meet with an accident while driving in heavy traffic and invite disaster.

3. Confidence Level

You cannot jump in the swimming pool as you lack confidence. Likewise, people never attempt to speak in public even they have good oratory but lack the confidence to appear in front of a mass or gathering.

4. Fear to Embrace Change

Most of my friends did not accept the change in the working environment; even experts had designed new models. Instead, they wanted to stick to their old patterns. For example, I saw people working in the same bank branch for a couple of decades and never opted to change the place due to fear of embracing the change.

B) External Factors

The external environment is equally responsible for not adopting learning, such as the following.

1. Environment

If the climatic condition is inadequate, you cannot develop certain sports or athletic abilities. Therefore, our coaching camp was shifted to a newer place where temperature and humidity matched suitable for the workouts.

2. Bad Experience

You might be hesitant to learn horse riding again if you were thrown from the horseback when it becomes hostile.

3. Lack of Innovation

The rigid unprofessional old style of teaching methodology may not imbibe a pleasant experience in the youth today. They may always want to have the latest technology in their learnings.

4. Unwilling to Unlearn

My grandfather used to tell the story of a marriage. There was a marriage ceremony in India where the bride and groom take seven rounds around the fire. The father of the groom had a tamed cat. He hid the cat underneath a basket through which the cat cannot come out but breathe. After 20 years, the groom's son was also getting married, and somebody said, "First hide the cat!" Again after the next 20 years, his grandchildren were getting married, but there was no cat nearby. So, the marriage was canceled as there was no cat available. The cat was hidden because it may not come on the way to the bride and groom when they were taking seven rounds around the fire as it is believed that when a cat crosses the path, it is thought to be a bad omen.

So, unlearning unwanted things are also necessary to learn new things.

Remedies To Update Learning

We cannot keep the space with the time if we are not actively participating and keeping pace with the technology.

1.   Repetition Is the mother of Learning

You cannot do a particular thing, and there is no shortcut for learning new things or new learning. For instance, you have to practice hours together for learning typing, swimming, cycling, driving, or boating. Moreover, things are unknown unless it achieves auto-pilot mode or stored in the subconscious mind. For instance, you are sometimes not conscious of applying a break or pushing the accelerator in traffic when driving.

2.   Follow the news to keep pace with current events

The media can be newspaper, radio, television, but it may help keep a good pace with current events or affairs. If you are not keeping pace with the current happenings, you may be thrown out like a wooden log in the river.

3.   Read books and articles or blogs

Reading is one of the most effective ways to learn new things. Many multimillionaires have explored the hidden potentials and gifted inventions and discoveries after reading books and articles.

4. Explore the internet to the fullest

The Internet has endless resources for learning. The abundance of information is increasing daily, and there is no limit to learning from online sites. There are thousands of institutes on specific education. Join the courses and learn on a daily basis.

5. Learn, implement and teach

When you have learned specific skills or hacks, apply them in your daily life and teach them to the target audience so that they are better retained in your mind and may be beneficial to the community, and the whole process may also become the source of income.

Key Take Away

1. To live a life without continuous learning is perishable status.

2. Continuous learning is self-motivated persistence in acquiring knowledge to reach the fullest potential of an individual.

Chapter Twelve: Skills Are Cheap, but Passions Are Priceless

"I was prepared to die with blood in my boots for 1500 meters race!"

-Sebastian Coe

Every living being learns from the experience. Even animals learn from previous experience. For example, whenever you have bitten the street dog entering your house because the dog is hungry and wants to eat something, he runs away when he sees you after entering your home because he fears that you may hit him again with the rod.

A generalized condition of your behavior happens with the repeated incidents in the past. We are well versed with the experiences of Russian psychologist[6] Ivan Pavlov who experimented on cats and dogs. Whenever food was served to the dog, he rang the bell. He could see the saliva from the dog's mouth because he had connected a device with a transparent tube to the dog's throat. At every incident, the dog salivated when food was served. It was repeated several times, and one day he saw that he rang the bell without food, the dog salivated. The animal had automatically trained his mind and assumed that there is food whenever there is a bell sound.

------

[6] Source: www.simplypsychology.org

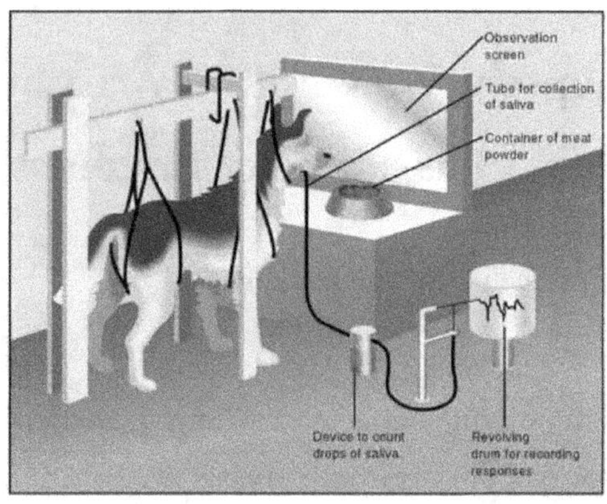

We as a human have some good or bad experiences in the past. We do not forget damaging or destructing incidents which have taken place in the past. You change the behavior on the basis of your past experience. For example, one of our neighbors left eating tobacco because his elder brother died of cancer as he was eating tobacco for several years. He was also consuming tobacco, but he survived because he thought he might die of cancer just like his brother.

The Choices You Make

I never touched the naked electrical wire after the incident of getting an electrical shock during my childhood. I adopted fasting because I had seen that my grandfather was doing so and lived for 99 years without medicines. I never repeated tearing off pages of my books during my school days because my father had locked me inside the room for several hours.

The book 'Food That Harms, The Food That heals' gave me a lot of knowledge, but I could choose my foods as some of them were the cause of my upset stomach. Like food, we have certain life incidents that control our specific behavior as we have faced the consequences. Whether the internal change is due to the effects of the excellent or external environment that has changed your behavior patterns, you may not accept yourself as less than the best version of yourself.

Why The Unstoppable

You are traveling abroad in the aircraft at 30000 feet height, and the crew tells you to jump from the plane with a parachute; you may think twice and refrain from jumping. But if the pilot declares that the aircraft has caught fire and there are no chances of survival, so jump out of the helicopter with your parachute. Although you may be fearing that parachute may open or not but you will prefer to jump. Your 'why' is much more critical than 'how.'

You may learn specific skills to do your piece of job you have undertaken, and there is no doubt that the particular skill will make your job very easy. The skills are the right kind of instruments to make your task easy. For instance, I want to plant a tree and start digging with Knife, but you are doing the same thing near the place, but you have a plow. You can turn up earth very quickly because you have a better instrument than I have. But if you do not have a passion for digging, you cannot have a fruitful result. If I have passion in my mind that I want to plant one hundred trees so that more people can get oxygen and earth may have a better place, nothing can stop me from digging with even improper instruments.

The more significant part of your work has resulted in a successful outcome if you love to do what you want to do. You can never be satisfied even if you reach your goal if you do not like to do what you do. One of my friend's son was never happy when he finished his medical degree when he passed out because he loved being an engineer. He joined medical college because his father could not become a doctor, and he wanted to make his son a doctor.

Passion is priceless irrespective of whether you possess a generic skill or niche skill. It is because emphasis promotes more involvement on the part of the individual concerned. The skills without passion will not help you stand out from the rest. On the contrary, it is passion coupled with skills that allows you to scale up.

Key Take Away
1. People with great passion can make the impossible happen.
2. Make your passion your pay-check

Chapter Thirteen: The Best Version of Yourself

"To be yourself in a world that is constantly trying to make you something else is the greatest accomplishment."

-Ralph Waldo Emerson

If you think that you have brushed your teeth and are shining or have worn perfect clothes after your bathe, are you the best version of yourself? Somebody may fall in love after seeing your hairstyle or the way you walk, but the physical appearance has only one-fourth importance of total aspects. You must have seen an example of an affluent girl falling in love with a poor boy or even her driver. It is not the only aspect that may be responsible for your traction. There are other aspects like mental, emotional, or spiritual.

The meaning of the best version has to be understood first. What does it mean by the best version? The best version of yourself cannot be the best version of somebody else. You may be surprised when interviews are conducted for a higher level of posts in corporate sectors. The person who has undergone training in leadership and entrepreneurship generally knows how to lead an organization. He is a master in the management of human resources, accounting, marketing, etc. What other types of skills have to be tested? I remember an interview of such a higher post when I was working as an official in one of the branches of the largest refinery; the qualified person was asked to bring her wife as a part of the interview process where his wife was asked few general questions.

As I had developed an intimate relationship with one of the general managers of the organization, I frankly asked when the person cooked product and familiar with almost all the fields, what kind of questions are asked in the interview? Since he was part of the interview process, he said that only one following question is asked in the discussion,

"What was the biggest failure in your life, and how could you overcome it? Narrate within the next 30 minutes. He said, "With one single question, we can judge his intelligence scale, mental ability, emotional stability, and spiritual quotient. Again I asked, but why the interview of his wife is required? He said with a great sense of humor, "If you are able to control your wife, you can control the whole world!" In fact, it is one of the interview techniques in which his relationship aspect is measured.

Rational Intelligence

When we say that someone is intelligent, we usually refer to their rational intelligence or the cognitive capacities that are tangible, measurable, and serve as the basis of most of our decisions.

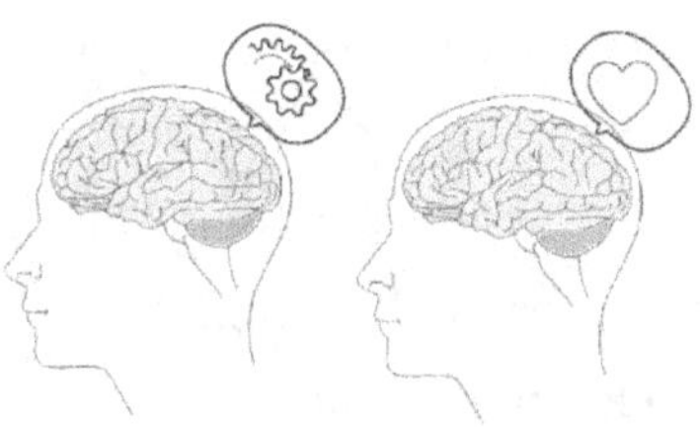

Emotional intelligence represents the capacity to join emotion and rationality: using emotions to facilitate reason and intelligently think about them. To be a successful person, one must have both emotional and social competencies. Individuals who have good emotional intelligence tend to be more successful and go further in their life. Sometimes, due to fame, position, and power, the ego is inflated like a hot air balloon. Therefore, emotional intelligence becomes a prime factor in managing his expectations and realities into a positive expected Value outcome; otherwise, he may get setback from the position or status he has achieved.

Power of Resilience

Resilience is the capacity or the ability of a person to recover from a problematic situation and sustain toughness like elastic. Resilience is the psychological quality that allows one to be knocked down by life's adversities and come back at least as strong as before. Rather than letting difficulties, traumatic events, or failure overcome them and drain their resolve, highly resilient people find a way to change course, emotionally heal, and continue moving toward their goals.

The essential factors for such resilience are morality, creativity, flexibility, passion, positive attitude, self-confidence, forgiveness, and a sense of humor. When the person develops the power of resilience, he becomes proactive. Strength is to overcome difficult situations, to learn from them, and to be able to change in a positive experience. If you cannot even manage your emotions, how can you manage the emotions of others? You may confront certain situations and deal with friends, relatives, or even a group of people you lead. A case was depicted on a real story in a recent movie where a young girl was recruited as the first woman pilot. There was no separate toilet or bathroom for ladies. How can she change the clothes when she has to share the barrack with her male counterparts? But she found the way and succeeded.

Raquel Caballero, a TED talk speaker, has given few imperative techniques as an outcome of her own experience.

She says to start working on your emotions. Stop ruminating and stop negative obsessive thoughts and start observing yourself. Convert negative emotions into positive experiences. In fact, emotions are not positive or negative. It depends upon you the way you handle it. The key is how you manage them effectively to your benefit.

Share your message with others. It is not an easy task, but it will give great relief. There is no single method, you may have your own strategies, but your achievement is reached with practice and rehearsals.

One of the world's leading experts in leadership development and emotional intelligence, Author and professor Richard Boyatzis [7] has developed expertise called Resonant Leadership that offers the tools to become the leader you want to be, including exercises to reassess valuable and effective techniques.

Key Take Away

1. Find your own method to manage your emotions, and you can be the best version of yourself.

2. Just like other common skills, you can master resilience by practice or rehearsal.

---

[7] Source: instituteofcoaching.org

Chapter Fourteen: Balance Your Pain and Pleasure

"The greatest pleasure in life is doing what people say you cannot do."

-Walter Bagehot

The pain-pleasure principle lies at the core of everything you do in everyday life. Your belief and value systems are built upon this principle. Your habits are built on the subject principle. Every decision you make in life is solely dependent on either pain or pleasure. Your behavior or action is based on your experience of joy and pain.

Past Experience of Pain and Pleasure

Consider the example of a lion in the circus. The lion is given pain by a hunter, even sometimes charged with minor electrical current. He is molded for particular actions or behavior with constant pains. The lion wants to avoid the pain, and therefore it does the determined activity by the trainer. With the previous experience of unbearable pain, it just obeys the command.

The experience of humans is also like other animals. His pains of the past which have given emotions of anger, hurt, stress, anxiety, overwhelm, frustration, depression, etc., have already made marks in the subconscious mind. Therefore, his present behavior or action is derived accordingly. But, on the other hand, his pleasant experiences of the past resulted in the emotions of

92

happiness, joy, enthusiasm, curiosity, love, gratitude, excitement, etc. are definitely responsible for his current thought process and actions.

Role Of Central Nervous System

When I put my finger in the electrical plug during my early childhood, it gave me a jerk. I was not sure what happened. So again, I checked with a thin iron rod; still, it gave me a shock. Later on, my teacher explained to me that electrical current passes through metal. During my master's in psychology, I studied that when electrical current is passed through our body, which is also a good conductor of electricity, it reaches the central nervous system after quickly traveling through thousands of neurons from one to another. Neurons or nerve cells are the primary components of the nervous system. They send and receive information in the form of electrical signals from the sensory organs, facilitating communication with the brain. The constant chatting between body and brain ultimately decides which signs are good and which are bad. In other words, which experiences are pleasant and which such experiences are painful. Like every other cell, neurons have a cell body, often referred to as the soma containing the nucleus. Various branches or finger-like structures extend from opposite sides of the soma. An axon is a more extended protrusion, while dendrites are the smaller branch-like structures on the other side of the soma.

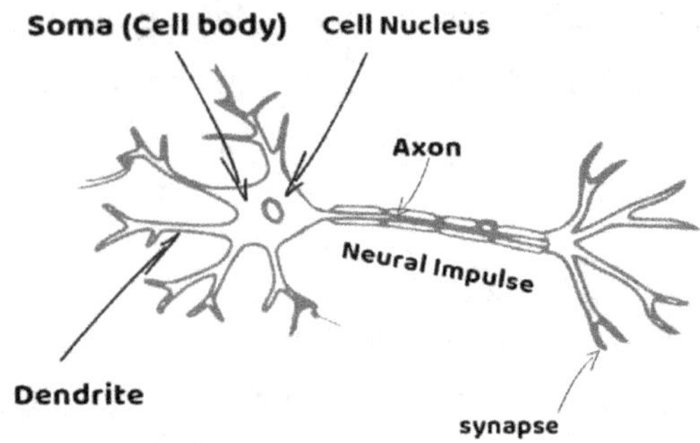

Neuro Transmission

Neurotransmission is the process by which the axon terminal of a neuron releases signaling molecules (neurotransmitters). They bind to and react with the receptors on the dendrites of another neuron (the postsynaptic neuron) a short distance away. Some neurons can release more than one neurotransmitter simultaneously, the other being a co-transmitter, to provide the stabilizing negative feedback required for meaningful encoding in the absence of inhibitory interneurons.

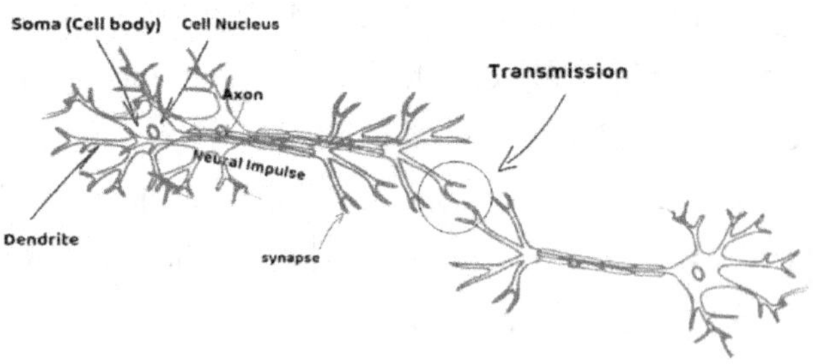

The transmission process is speedy as compared to the speed of blood flow, with some myelinated neurons conducting at speeds up to 120 m/s (432 km/h or 275 mph). You can imagine the speed of neurotransmission by comparing it to an athlete who runs the 100 meters within 10 seconds. You suppose that this transmission is almost ten times the speed of an athlete.

I, later on, realized after my Neuro-Linguistic Programming training how I was able to remove my hand so quickly from a live electrical point to nullify the counter effect of the shock. It is because the brain is believed to possess such 86 billion neurons on average. And therefore, the complex process of such transmission is possible.

Pain And Pleasure Psychology

People move toward pleasure because they find happiness, and they move away from pain because they are not happy with suffering. It is literally the whole sum of the psychology of why people do things they do.

Our mind constantly works day and night without rest to weigh out the pain and pleasure of every effort we make. So it is really working on getting the cause benefitting analysis and making efforts to maximize the satisfaction and minimize the pain. Even you try to kill mosquito with your hand hitting your forehead even when you are sleeping because your mind, mainly subconscious mind, is working. So it is simple in every piece of behavior.

I studied in clinical psychology that If one can control the pleasure and pain of a person, one can get anything done from the person. We have generally understood pain and pleasure in broad terms, and we usually narrow it down to physical pain and physical pleasure. But as a matter of fact, any easiness or uneasiness is a concern of pleasure or pain principle respectively. You must have felt when you are with your good friends, things turn up to the pleasure principle and say, for instance, it definitely turns to the pain principle when you have been forced to achieve some target in your office by your boss. However, a threshold can vary from person to person.

Another example of pleasure and pain you must have experienced during public speaking. When you have to present yourself in front of an audience, you may perceive the pain that you may forget the lines, and the public may insult you. But when you repeatedly speak in practice, your pain vanishes. Concerning pleasure, one experience that when you provide great values and people transform their lives, the positive feelings will perceive the pleasure state.

Exemptions

Sometimes some of the social workers suffer pain to give pleasure to other people. However, in another way, they have pleasure of minimizing the pain of others.

Key Take Away

1. Psychologically, it is believed that you can perform any task twice more to avoid the pain than to gain pleasure.

2. There is nothing like unselfish behavior.

Chapter Fifteen: Emotional traits transient

"Never let negative emotions influence your faith."

-Dr. Jacinta Mpalyenkana, PhD, MBA

Human is emotional wellbeing. The effect of the internal or external environment is crucial for individual development. The energy may get blocked or released as an aftereffect of emotion. It depends upon personal maturity. One may burst into tears after watching a social drama in a movie or episode of a serial on television, and other individuals may laugh at the incident. You may laugh after a witty joke of a stand-up comedian, but I may not even smile. Your happiness or pain depends upon your thought process, which seriously you take an incident, whether on social media or an actual event in front of your eyes.

Emotional manipulators dangerous

It depends upon your personality traits who deeply the manipulators affect you. An emotional manipulator, in one way, is so toxic that you may sometime do not notice your act or the consequences may be very much hazardous to your health or critical to managing your behavior. The manipulator is always craving the attention of people. A person may complain about the small piece of the task he does not want to undergo so that he has to climb the mountain. Things are sometimes far away from the truth, and therefore manipulator tries to twist the fact and prove you wrong by convincing you according to their perception. With aggression and information overload, they relentlessly pressurize you with a sense of urgency. An emotional manipulator is always ready to turn something positive into something negative. They are experts at using your conscience against you, prompting you to feel guilty even when you have done nothing wrong. They may not take things seriously but also try to encourage them to listen to them and act positively on their intentions.

Emotional Personality Disorders

An emotionally affected person may constantly seek attention and speak dramatically expressive words to gain the sympathy of others; however, such persons can easily be influenced if handled intelligently. In this subject affair, emotions may be shallow, rapid, dramatic, and sometimes sexually provocative since the emotional vampires are so strong that they may drastically affect the human psychosomatic structure. It is also a fact that positive emotions show joy and happiness as they release hormones responsible for strengthening the immune system. But at the same time, it may also be found that negative emotions may have the opposite effect. They may weaken the immune system, making your body more prone to illness.

Physical Disorders

Emotional distress damages a person physically in such a way that the victim may have serious consequences. For example, emotional stress may cause a stroke or lead to blood urination problems called UTI or urinal tract infections. A person who has been affected may hardly assimilate external events. The resultant resentment or anger may cause dramatic consequences. In fact, others may not be aware of individual sadness causing a "burning" sensation or irritation. Sudden pain in the lower left side of the abdomen, called diverticulitis symptoms, is the most common. Other symptoms may include abdominal pain, nausea, vomiting, fever, bloating, or constipation. Emotion for a prolonged time may invite disorders like stroke, eye problems, and even epilepsy. It is a pretty severe affair as emotional instability results in damage to the hippocampus, a brain area involved in learning and memory ability. Emotional pains are stored in the body. The wounds may not be visible, but sometimes the effect can be perceived through tears in the eyes. The emotionally affected person may constantly feel weak and have fatigue.

Mental Disorders

The overall subject affairs may significantly affect the relationships and limit social activities at the workplace and home. Moreover, the continuous effects may bridge the disorders like paranoid personality disorder, schizoid personality disorder, narcissistic personality disorder, or obsessive-compulsive personality disorder. In case of any signs or symptoms of a personality disorder, it is advisable to see a mental health professional. If the unusual behavior is untreated, personality disorders can cause significant problems in your life that may get worse without treatment.

According to Kendra Cherry, MS, an author, educational consultant, and speaker focused on helping students learn about psychology. There are six types of basic emotions and their effects on human behavior.

i. Happiness

Out of all the different emotions, happiness tends to be the one that people strive for the most. Happiness is often defined as a pleasant emotional state characterized by feelings of contentment, joy, gratification, satisfaction, and well-being.

Research on happiness has increased significantly since the 1960s within several disciplines, including psychology, known as positive psychology. This type of emotion is sometimes expressed through:

Facial expressions: such as smiling

Body language: such as a relaxed stance

The tone of voice: an upbeat, pleasant way of speaking

While happiness is considered one of the basic human emotions, the things we think will create happiness tend to be heavily influenced by culture. For example, pop culture influences tend to emphasize that attaining certain items such as buying a home or having a high-paying job will result in happiness.

The realities of what contributes to happiness are often much more complex and more highly individualized.2□ People have long believed that happiness and health were connected, and research has supported the idea that joy can play a role in both physical and mental health.

Happiness has been linked to a variety of outcomes, including increased longevity and increased marital satisfaction.3□ Conversely, unhappiness has been linked to a variety of poor health outcomes.

Stress, anxiety, depression, and loneliness, for example, have been linked to things such as lowered immunity, increased inflammation, and decreased life expectancy.

ii. Sadness

Sadness is another type of emotion often defined as a transient emotional state characterized by a feeling of disappointment, grief, hopelessness, disinterest, and dampened mood.

Like other emotions, sadness is something that all people experience from time to time. However, in some cases, people can experience prolonged and severe periods of sadness that can turn into depression. Sadness can be expressed in many ways, including:

- Crying
- Dampened mood
- Lethargy

- Quietness
- Withdrawal from others

The type and severity of sadness can vary depending upon the root cause, and how people cope with such feelings can also differ.

Sadness can often lead people to engage in coping mechanisms such as avoiding other people, self-medicating, and ruminating on negative thoughts. Unfortunately, such behaviors can actually exacerbate feelings of sadness and prolong the duration of the emotion.

iii. **Fear**

Fear is a powerful emotion that can also play an essential role in survival. When you face some sort of danger and experience fear, you go through what is known as the fight or flight response.

Your muscles become tense, your heart rate and respiration increase, and your mind become more alert, priming your body to either run from the danger or stand and fight.

This response helps ensure that you are ready to deal with threats in your environment effectively. Expressions of this type of emotion can include:

Facial expressions: such as widening the eyes and pulling back the chin

Body language: attempts to hide or flee from the threat

Physiological reactions: such as rapid breathing and heartbeat

Of course, not everyone experiences fear in the same way. Some people may be more sensitive to stress, and certain situations or objects may be more likely to trigger this emotion.

Fear is the emotional response to an immediate threat. However, we can also develop a similar reaction to anticipated threats or even our thoughts about potential dangers, and this is what we generally think of as anxiety. Social anxiety, for example, involves an anticipated fear of social situations.

Some people, on the other hand, actually seek out fear-provoking situations. For example, extreme sports and other thrills can be fear-inducing, but some people seem to thrive and even enjoy such feelings.

Repeated exposure to a fearful object or situation can lead to familiarity and acclimation, reducing feelings of fear and anxiety.

This is the idea behind exposure therapy, in which people are steadily exposed to the things that frighten them in a controlled and safe manner. Eventually, feelings of fear begin to decrease.

iv. **Disgust**

Disgust is another of the original six basic emotions described by Eckman. Disgust can be exhibited in different ways, including:

Body language: turning away from the object of disgust

Physical reactions: such as vomiting or retching

Facial expressions: such as wrinkling the nose and curling the upper lip

This sense of disgust can originate from many things, including an unpleasant taste, sight, or smell. Researchers believe that this emotion evolved as a reaction to foods that might be harmful or fatal. When people smell or taste foods that have gone bad, disgust is a typical reaction.

Poor hygiene, infection, blood, rot, and death can also trigger a disgust response. It may be the body's way of avoiding things that may carry transmittable diseases.

People can also experience moral disgust when they observe others engaging in behaviors that they find distasteful, immoral, or evil.

v. **Anger**

Anger can be a compelling emotion characterized by feelings of hostility, agitation, frustration, and antagonism towards others. Like fear, anger can play a part in your body's fight or flight response.

When a threat generates feelings of anger, you may be inclined to fend off the danger and protect yourself. But, instead, anger is often displayed through:

Facial expressions: such as frowning or glaring

Body language: such as taking a solid stance or turning away

The tone of voice: such as speaking gruffly or yelling

Physiological responses: such as sweating or turning red

Aggressive behaviors: such as hitting, kicking, or throwing objects

While anger is often thought of as a negative emotion, it can sometimes be a good thing. It can be constructive in helping clarify your needs in a relationship, and it can also motivate you to take action and find solutions to items that are bothering you.

However, anger can become a problem when it is excessive or expressed in unhealthy, dangerous, or harmful ways. Uncontrolled anger can quickly turn to aggression, abuse, or violence.

This type of emotion can have both mental and physical consequences. For example, unchecked anger can make it difficult to make rational decisions and even impact your physical health.

Anger has been linked to coronary heart diseases and diabetes. It has also been linked to behaviors that pose health risks, such as aggressive driving, alcohol consumption, and smoking.

vi. **Surprise**

Surprise is another one of the six basic types of human emotions originally described by Eckman. Shock is usually relatively brief and is characterized by a physiological startle response following something unexpected.

This type of emotion can be positive, negative, or neutral. An unpleasant surprise, for example, might involve someone jumping out from behind a tree and scaring you as you walk to your car at night.

An example of a pleasant surprise would be arriving home to find that your closest friends have gathered to celebrate your birthday. Wonder is often characterized by: Facial expressions: such as raising the brows, widening the eyes, and opening the mouth

Physical responses: such as jumping back

Verbal reactions: such as yelling, screaming, or gasping

Surprise is another type of emotion that can trigger a fight or flight response. When startled, people may experience a burst of adrenaline that helps prepare the body to either fight or flee.□

Surprise can have significant effects on human behavior. For example, research has shown that people tend to notice surprising events disproportionately.

This is why dramatic and unusual events in the news tend to stand out in memory more than others. Research has also found that people tend to be more swayed by surprising arguments and learn more from incredible information.

> **Key Take Away**
>
> 1. It is your responsibility for your feelings, emotions, and behavior which are the outcome of your practices and not others.
>
> 2. Emotional intelligence can play a vital role as the most potent weapon in our armory.

Chapter Sixteen: Amount of Sleep

"I prefer insomnia to anesthesia."

-Antonio Tabucchi

A sound sleep is essential, just like any other basic needs in human life like food or water. The lack of sleep may shorten life. Through statistics, it has been observed that those who have slept for 5 hours a day have lived less by a decade than individuals who slept for 7 hours a day. The level of testosterone found in the former was lesser for his counterpart, who was senior by ten years. This is equally applicable to males and females. Sleep has a catastrophic impact on health and wellness. Impairment of reproductive organs was observed in the female who had a lack of sleep.

Impact of Sleep on Learning

It was experienced that proper sleep is necessary before learning and also after learning for better retention. The memory is drastically affected due to lack of sleep. The brain acts just like a sponge full of water. If you do not sleep properly, the elements of learning are not absorbed.

Two groups of people experimented, where one group was allowed to sleep correctly, and the other group was deprived of sleep. When an MRI scan was done for both groups, surprising results were observed in both groups. Almost 40% of the memory deficit was found for the group deprived of sleep compared to the group who slept adequately. This is a matter of concern even for children because I will never like it if my child will fail an examination due to learning disabilities or poor memory retention and spoil his whole career just for lack of sleep. I never preferred computers with lesser memory because they bounced back the intake of a new file. How can I afford less storage in my brain for less memory retention experience due to fewer hours of sleep! Proper sleep converts a large amount of short-term memories to long-term memories in adequate quantity.

Aging And Dementia

The constant deprivation of sleep may cause different types of disorders. It may lead to Alzheimer's disease too. Is it advisable to take sleeping and other related drugs and treat Alzheimer's or central neurocognitive disorders like Dementia? It is always better to take more water to treat thicker blood than the deadly side effect of pills to treat the same with medications. In the same way, if the nutritional quality of sleep is made a habit, you are saved from drugs and free from these deadly diseases.

Sleep And Cardiovascular System

Improper sleeping experience has a nasty effect on cardiovascular systems too. In a TED talk by Matt Walker, it was described that a global experiment performed on 1.6 billion people across 70 countries twice a year, and it's called daylight saving time. Now, when we lose one hour of sleep in the spring, we see a subsequent 24-percent increase in heart attacks that following day. Conversely, when we gain an hour of sleep in the autumn, we see a 21-percent reduction in heart attacks. Isn't that incredible? And you see exactly the same profile for car crashes, road traffic accidents, even suicide rates.

Sleep And DNA Genetic Code

In his further explanation, Walker also explained the consequences of the ill effect of improper sleep on DNA. Lack of sleep will even erode the very fabric of biological life itself, your DNA genetic code. So here in this study, they took a group of healthy adults, and they limited them to six hours of sleep a night for one week. Then they measured the change in their gene activity profile relative to when those same individuals were getting a total of eight hours of sleep a night. And there were two critical findings. First, a sizable and significant 711 genes were distorted in their activity, caused by a lack of sleep. The second result shows that about half of the genes were increased in their movement, and the other half were decreased.

Now those genes that were switched off by a lack of sleep were genes associated with your immune system, so once again, you can see that immune deficiency. In contrast, those genes that were upregulated or increased by way of a lack of sleep were genes associated with the promotion of tumors, genes related to long-term chronic inflammation within the body, and genes related to stress, and, as a consequence, cardiovascular disease.

There is simply no aspect of your wellness that can retreat at the sign of sleep deprivation and get away unscathed. It's rather like a broken water pipe in your home. Sleep loss will leak down into every nook and cranny of your physiology, even tampering with the very DNA nucleic alphabet that spells out your daily health narrative.

Finally, he gave two pieces of advice for sleep.

1.   The first is regularity.

Go to bed simultaneously, wake up at the same time, no matter whether it's the weekday or the weekend. Regularity is king, and it will anchor your sleep and improve the quantity and the quality of that sleep.

2.   Keep Your Room cool.

Your body needs to drop its core temperature by about two to three degrees Fahrenheit to initiate sleep and then to stay asleep, and it's the reason you will always find it easier to fall asleep in a room that's too cold than too hot. So aim for a bedroom temperature of around 65 degrees or about 18 degrees Celsius. That's going to be optimal for the sleep of most people.

Key Take Away

1.   Shorten your sleep and shorten your life.
2.   Sleep is not a luxury but a non-negotiable biological necessity.

Chapter Seventeen: Limited Resources or Unlimited Resourcefulness

"If you always put a limit on everything you do, physical or anything else. It will spread into your work and your life. There are no limits. There are only plateaus, and you must not stay there; you must go beyond them."

-Bruce Lee

Being resourceful means utilizing the readily available supplies, tools, and information sources that we have. We start blaming the lack of resources and procrastinate, although resources are available to us. I used to tell my mentor that, "I am too young to practice meditation." The subject practice should be started at the age of 12 years. One of my friends did not start his business, saying that he did not have enough capital. One of my old friends wrote me that he wished he could be an author, but he did not have time. There number of excuses for breaking the ice, but those who want to do it can do so in any prevailing situation.

Seeds of Flowers

I heard a story about an older man who proceeded for a religious tour and called his three sons. He offered some seeds of flowers and said, these are essential resources for you, and I want them in return when I come back from the tour. So, he gave three bags of seeds to each of their sons and left for the tour.

When he returned after three whole years, he enquired about the seeds issued to them. Elder son replied,

"The moment you left, I kept the seeds in our treasury safely so that I could preserve them to hand them over to you."

The tears were almost to shade from the eyes of the man, but he did not react.

When he asked the middle son what he had done with the seeds, he replied,

"I am a businessman; I sold it to market, and I will just now purchase the seeds in equal quantity just now so that I can give you the fresh seeds in return."

Tears again shaded from the father's eyes but did not speak anything and proceeded to the youngest son.

The youngest son responded in the following manners,

"Dear father, I do not have to say anything about the seed, but you have to accompany me to the backside yards with me."

The father's eyes were full of tears but with joy and satisfaction when he saw the garden full of flowers.

Every son used the resources as per their mentality and thoughts, but the reactions were different.

Alexander Graham Bell

American inventor Alexander Graham Bell was hard of hearing but invented the telephone. He could have said, "I want to invent an instrument that can connect two human beings, but I am hard of hearing and cannot do it!" In fact, he developed a system that converted voice into text, and he did not even have fully functional instruments. At every moment, he faced challenges. Technology was not feasible. He even sold his stocks and savings for investing in his experiments. Nevertheless, he contributed to research into the worldwide 'Hello Effect' that provided practical applications later in our present time.

Bruce Lee

Bruce Lee, the martial artist, and actor dramatically influenced and changed martial arts, but very few people knew that his one leg was shorter than the other one. Still, he made the shorter leg his lethal weapon as an additional advantage and defeated the opponent. One of the challenges of Bruce Lee was nearsighted. His bad eyesight is one reason he appreciated Wing Chun's contact style of movement because he could rely more on touch than sight. Due to his bad eyesight, Bruce Lee was one of the first people to try contact lenses.

Kapil Dev

Indian skipper Kapil Dev wrote in his biography. He has introduced to the Indian coach as a fast bowler. However, his coach said, "There is no fast bowler in India!" He could have taken it as his limitation, but he took these negative words as a challenge. India could see the glimpses of winning the 1983 world cup as his thrilling inning as a bowler but smashing 16 boundaries and six sixes during his knock of 175 runs.

Some find excuses, and some find reasons. Resourcefulness is the ability to find answers to existing questions and overcome challenges. The true warrior always accepts the challenge and believes that he does not know everything but knows enough. He learns from people and situations. Therefore, he continuously optimizes the recourses available to him.

The most successful people in the world use their resourcefulness on a daily basis, even when the number of challenges. They make resourcefulness a part of your daily mindset, and they are always doing more with fewer recourses.

Key Take Away

1. "It's not the lack of resources that cause failure; it's the lack of resourcefulness that causes failure."-Tony Robbins

2. "When you can't change the direction of the wind — adjust your sails"-H. Jackson Brown, Jr.

Chapter Eighteen: Mirror Neurons: Causing Change Within Others

"Yesterday I was clever, so I wanted to change the world. Today I am wise, so I am changing myself."

-Rumi

Have you any time thought about why you cry while watching a tragedy seen in a movie? Have you noticed why you laugh while watching the comedy show? The mirror neurons which are activated in your brain are responsible for the subject's reaction.

What Is Mirror Neuron?

A mirror neuron is a neuron that fires both when an animal acts and when the animal observes the same action performed by another. Thus, the neuron "mirrors" the behavior of the other, as though the observer were itself acting. Such neurons have been directly observed in human and primate species and birds. Mirror neurons are found in the inferior frontal cortex and superior Parietal lobe of the human brain.

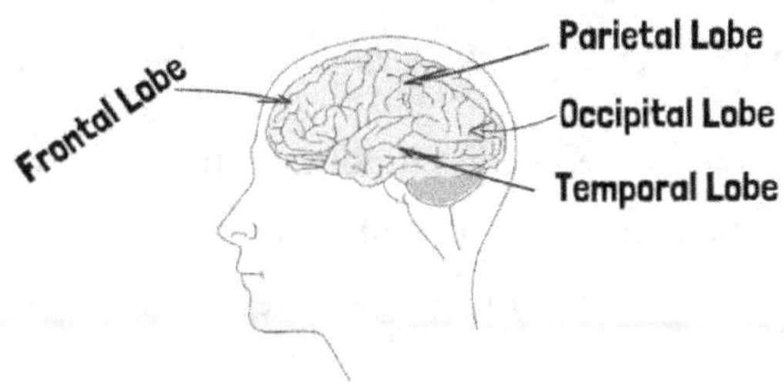

The striking implication of mirror neurons is that the same brain region that controls action also supports perception. If observing behavior occurs in the same area as behaving, social interaction would play a prominent role in cognition.

Behavior Of Monkeys

I have to share a true story of monkeys which suddenly arrived in my village 45 years ago. It is a real story when I was studying in school. Four monkeys stayed almost for one year in the town; one was male, one was female, and two were young. We used to throw some food at them, and they instantly caught and ate them. For example, when we threw bananas, the young ones did not know how to open the banana. When we used to peel the banana, the monkeys followed and ate like men. I was astonished by this learning activity, but I knew in detail later on during my master's in psychology.

The work done with monkeys in Rizzolatti's lab gave a name to the multitasking mental cells that make this possible. Mirror neurons fire when monkeys break peanuts in their hands when they see others break peanuts — even when, in total darkness, they merely hear peanuts being broken. "It's almost like the monkey is watching his action reflected by the mirror."

Mirror neurons haven't been pinpointed in people with the same precision that electrodes can identify them in monkeys. Still, several recent functional imaging studies support a social side to human cognition, with which people internally replay the actions they view in another before acting themselves.

In a 2003 study in the Proceedings of the National Academy of Sciences[8], a research team that included Iacoboni found that imitating and observing facial expressions activated the same regions of the brain. In addition, a study in science a year later showed activity in similar neural areas whether a subject experienced a painful stimulus or observed a loved one receiving the same shock. To many researchers, these and similar findings suggest that mirror neurons play a significant role in empathy.

Quality Of Humaneness

You must have observed, especially when you are with your young child, that the child starts crying when you make an angry face. But when you smile or laugh, your child starts laughing just like you. So, when you have certain acts of happiness or angriness, the observer's mirror neurons are activated, and signal to motor neurons and subject behavior is manifested. So it clearly means that there is an effect of negativity and positivity in others' brain and their relative behavior.

I was surprised while traveling in train during a halt for five minutes in a station when my wife started picking up fruits thrown on the platform from a basket of vendors due to the heavy rush of passengers. She was handing over each piece to

____

[8] Source: www.psychologicalscience.org

him after leaving her baggage with me. She was so empathic during the situation that she almost wept. During that incident, I did not feel much, maybe, due to nerve damage caused by the parade and protruding nails in my shoes to my brain as I was a soldier.

Sympathy And Empathy

Sympathy, constructed from the Greek[9] syn, meaning "together," and pathos, referring to feeling or emotion, is used when one person shares the senses. For example, one experiences sadness when someone close is experiencing grief or loss. Empathy is a newer word also related to "pathos." It differs from sympathy in implying greater emotional distance. With empathy, you can imagine or understand how someone might feel without necessarily having those feelings yourself.

Eye Contacts and Smiles

You never know the effects of your eye contact or smile you have given to your near and dear ones or strangers. Always put your legs in the shoes of others. Your pains are not the pains of others. You may be narrating the story of the death of your relative, but the person in conversation with you might not be interested as he or she may be having unbearable pain in his tooth. If you want to help others or build your community, you can always have a smile on your face with intense eye contact. It will have a

---

[9] Source: www.merriam-webster.com

profound effect on others. We can build the good versions of people coming into our connection and make the earth a better place for each other and live happy and peaceful lives.

Key Take Away

1. Prefer empathy over sympathy because empathy fuels connection while sympathy drives disconnection.

2. A smile is an act of compassion.

Chapter Nineteen: Connect to Your Inner Self

"You are who you are when nobody's watching."

-Stephen Fry

Human has four significant aspects of being physical, mental, emotional, and spiritual. Generally speaking, in most cases, we consider physical elements and then decide our progress. It means we are giving importance to 25 % of the total possibilities. Therefore, we are deprived of the rest of 75% possibilities. When we present ourselves to others, we go by appearance. We apply cosmetics, oil, trim our hair, etc. But we forget the expression of our hidden abilities, reaction strength, and compassion inbuilt in ourselves. Still, generally, we do not sometimes utilize it during the whole course of our life span.

It can be explained more clearly through an example of the software and hardware of a computer. Suppose you have written a paragraph, and when you take the print, you find that there was a spelling mistake. If you try anything with your printer, you cannot change the printed material. You have to amend the document, save it and then print it. Our external appearance or physical well-being is just like a computer. Of course, just like a printer, it has also got the value, but you cannot have good results of your activities or behavior output without internal changes.

Internal growth is hidden and sometimes cannot be judged externally. The trees are good examples. Externally we see the beautiful structure of tree-like stems, branches, leaves, flowers, etc. But the leading cause responsible for standing and providing ample facilities lies in the roots. If the roots are not strong, any storm can destroy the tree. In the same way, human also has other aspects like mental toughness, emotional stability, and spiritual existence as his important characteristics to withstand possible storms in real life.

If you are internally strong, it reflects in the outside world. One of my mentors always said, "Open your mouth, and I will tell you about your image." Your word is coming out of your mouth the way you think. If your thoughts are positive, you speak positively. But your thoughts are negative; you cannot expect the word to be positive and cannot predict things to happen in the desired manner.

In contrast to the outer self, the inner self is about what can't be seen externally. Your feelings, intuition, values, beliefs, personality, thoughts, fantasies, desire, and purpose are hidden inside you, just like that of the roots of a tree. A robust inner self means that you cope well with your emotions, are self-aware, have clarity and a good sense of your values, and feel a profound purpose in life.

How To Connect to Inner Self

You can be alive and worthy if you connect yourself internally. Be introverted when you are alone. Being self-centered is an ability that can define your personality. You inevitably miss the main person in your life if you are not connecting with your inner self. You can link internally in the following manner.

1.   Breathing Exercise

Our entire existence is dependent on breathing. Stop breathing, and your existence is finished. If the duration of your breathing is short, you may have a shorter life. But if you can live with a more extended period, your life can be longer. It is probably the best time to undergo breathing when you breathe a certain amount of air goes in your body through the lungs. When you breathe in, you extract the supply of Sulphur dioxide, Nitrous oxide, Ozone, Nitrogen dioxide, Iodine, etc., apart from oxygen. Oxygen is the main course for your existence. While you breathe out, you throw out carbon dioxide and an inevitable part of oxygen. Almost 5% of oxygen is retained in the body. The longer you breathe, the percentage may amount to be more in quantity.

To better regulate these resources available in the air, we need to do certain pranayama, yogic exercises, meditation, and mudras. Deep breathing in a silent climate, especially early morning, may give an added advantage. Sit in meditating posture. It may be on the ground or a chair too. Suppose you are not able to concentrate on breathing count your inhaling and exhaling, first in increasing order and then in decreasing manner. Observe your breath which you inhale from nose to deeper level at the abdomen and exhale from the abdomen to nose. Generally, it is the path from Ingla-Pingal to Nabhi and vice-versa. Inhaling, pause, and exhaling, spiritually called Purak, Kumbhak and Rachak, have generally specified timings. The waiting time should be double than the inhaling, and then the exhaling time should be almost four times than the inhaling for better retention of oxygen in the body.

2. Journaling

Journaling is nothing but writing in a journal or diary on a daily basis. It is a process of creating a shadow copy of messages happening or occurring inside your mind. The transparency of this exercise will make the quality more profound. It is the best way to record your thoughts and feelings. The journaling practice of my early days is now coming out as outlines of my books at present.

Journaling is considered the oldest form of self-help globally; it explores one's own thoughts, feelings, impulses, memories, goals, and hidden desires through written words. I observed during psychological studies that journaling is often prescribed by therapists, counselors, and spiritual mentors as a powerful way of developing more self-understanding and compassion.

Exploring uncomfortable emotions, incidents and facts can sometimes be challenging in all kinds of ways. Your little diary

(Darling I Always Remember You) may be a more prosperous, more fulfilling life to keep reading. It can be uplifting, and we can also feel like we're being scrubbed across the washboard of unpleasant history and wrung through the mangle of overwhelming emotion.

3. Yoga and Meditation

One of the most incredible options to get the internal positive energies flowing is to do yoga. You can personalize this practice to what you like and feel comfortable with. It is a widely accepted practice almost in all cultural and geographical setups.

Yoga is almost everything about learning and undergoing the magical movements of different parts of our body. It's a fantastic way to find balance in connecting the mind and inner self. The initial activities of the body part in the easiest way can be practice by Surya Namaskar. Later on, the wide range of yogic exercises can be extended from Hath yoga to Nauli Kriya. These beautiful techniques have the most significant advantage right from the purification of abdomen, body as a whole, to mind and soul.

Self-Empowerment

You are the powerhouse of your energies. Whatever is available in-universe is available in your body. Some individuals can generate plenty of energy from within, and some individuals can never understand the energy pond within. We have a hectic schedule in existing time with various activities whether it is fruitful for life or just passing the time without having any good benefits. Mindful exercise is needed how much time to be allotted to such activities. If a passion-driven life with a self-centered approach is evolved, life can differ from ordinary or average living style.

Chapter Twenty: Adapt to A Changed World

"Change is the law of life. And those who look only to the past or the present are certain to miss the future"

-John F Kennedy

Change is an ability to accept what you cannot control rather than what you can control. Change is always constant in our life. Resistance to change is the de-acceleration of our progress. If you do not accept the change, you fall prey to decay. When you have hindrance to changing situations, You worsen your abilities just like rotten iron. As the saying goes, the 'fittest will survive; if you escape the impact of change, you may elope gradually like dinosaurs.

Step Out of Comfort Zone

The leading cause for refraining from change is fear. It is always the false event appearing real. For example, when you are traveling on the train and all of a sudden somebody enters the compartment, you must have heard voices, "There is no place here, go to the next compartment!" You want to be more and more comfortable and do not want to be disturbed in an existing situation. The person who has entered stays back with a leap of faith despite trivial remarks, but after some time, you gradually start talking to him, and he becomes your companion.

The change may be planned like the working hours of your organization. You may have to get up a little early if the business hours are advanced for a couple of hours or unplanned, like changing the place of residence caught in a fire and household goods were destroyed beyond economical repair.

Denial And Acceptance Of Change

When the doctor declared that my brother, who was in one of the Air Defence Regiments in the Army, could not survive for a couple of years, I was in a denial state of change. Generally, the emotional pain lasts for few minutes, and definitely, the later time is the only reflection. I accepted the uncontrolled change and took him to our home place.

Some unplanned changes can be accepted by reading books and listening to podcasts or discourses from valuable dignitaries. With combinations of some of them, I took a master's course in psychology for two years to understand sclerosis in the brain and some of the curing techniques for subject ailment through abnormal psychology, simultaneously looking after my younger brother. The adopted change could increase the possibilities and hopes for my brother, who survived for the next 13 years.

Change Your Habits and Change Your Life

Some individuals adapt to bad habits like alcohol or drugs to compensate for the denial of unbearable tragedy or sudden incapacitation. But this is the wrong way of adaptation. Instead, the right ways may be related to fruitful readings.

Books are definitely the pathways for volunteer changes. However, the one thing I liked the most about book reading is a beautiful fact that you can never argue! Following three masterpieces made drastic positive changes in my life.

First is 'Million Dollar Habits" by Brian Tracy. The author thought process changed my life to form 21 new habits from progressive personal life to growing corporate job interactions.

The second is "5 am Club" by Robin Sharma. Changing the habit of a late-night owl to an early-rising bird made physical and mental fitness stronger for fighting day-to-day stresses.

The third one is "What to Say When You Talk to Yourself" by Dr. Shad Helmstetter. The book taught me how to accept, recognize, and need to change, change, and accept change for the betterment and universal affirmation.

Kintsugi Technique

It is a Japanese art of repairing broken pottery as a new work of art with gold. Thus, a unique piece of art is transformed into a new form or work with an adapted change in structure.

The name of the technique is derived from the words "Kin" (golden) and "tsugi" (joinery), which translate to mean "golden repair."

Just like the ceramic piece or the pottery, several human beings have cracks in their lives and sojourned to an emotional breakdown. Even though ceramic is not wasted and thrown away, how can valuable human life be neglected? The change you could make just like the golden filling in ceramic, you can adapt to the difference in their lives. You can never know how your efforts may transform them to live in their golden era.

5 Strategies for Adapting to Change

Career Resilience Coach Kathryn Sandford has given the following five strategies in Lifehack[10] to enable, adapt and successfully manage change in your life.

1.   Changing Your Mind-Set – Your Power Choice

"Progress is impossible without change, and those who cannot change their minds cannot change anything."

— George Bernard Shaw

We like to live our lives in our comfort zone. Our subconscious likes this because it is the "known." However, embracing change is stepping into the unknown, and our subconscious will do not like the "unknown." so it will resist.

Our fear and self-limiting beliefs will kick into action when we are faced with the disruptive consequences of change. There is no escaping the fact that change is a disruptor, and it feels uncomfortable and scary. However, it is our power of choice that enables us to activate positive change in our lives.

---

[10] Source: www.lifehack.org

We cannot control the events of change in our lives, but we can control how we react to these events' impact on our lives.

"Life is about choices. Some we regret, some we're proud of. Some will haunt us forever. The message: we are what we chose to be." — Graham Brown

The more you use your power of choice, and the more you focus your mindset on positively adapting to change, the more resilient you will be to dealing with the impact that change will bring to your life.

2. Find Meaning in Life

"Step out of your comfort zone. Comfort zones, where your unrealized dreams are buried, are the enemies of achievement. Leadership begins when you step outside your comfort zone."

— Roy T. Bennett

Knowing what is essential in your life gives you purpose and sets the direction of how you want to live your life. With a sense of purpose and meaning in life, you have clarity and focus, and both these elements are essential to you being able to successfully adapt and manage the impact of change in your life.

Having no purpose or meaning means that you tend to drift in life within the confines of your comfort zone. But conversely, purpose and meaning in life give you the courage to step out of your comfort zone – which is where you will find change and the opportunities it can offer to you.

3. Let Go of Your Regrets

The truth is unless you let go unless you forgive yourself, unless you forgive the situation unless you realize that the problem is over, you cannot move forward."

— Steve Maraboli

Regrets have a massive impact on how you respond to change and hold you back in life. So letting go of your guilt is key to you being able to move forward in life.

It is the events of change that present opportunities in life, so you may miss the present and future prospects if you are looking back at your past.

You cannot change what you did or did not do in the past so let it go. The only control you have now is to choose to live in your present and future life.

A great exercise to deal with regrets in life is to blow up a heap of balloons and, on each balloon, write a pang of guilt. Then, let the balloon go. Then, as the balloon drifts off, out loud, say goodbye to that regret.

A very simple but effective way of dealing with the pile of regrets you have collected in your lives.

4. Write a List of Scary Things to Do – Then Do Them

Change is scary, and it is all about stepping out of your comfort zone into the unknown. So, our subconscious needs to get familiar with us stepping out of a comfort zone and doing scary things. We want to train our subconscious to believe that stepping out of our comfort zone and doing difficult things is normal for us to do.

Make a list of scary things that you would like to do but have been too afraid to. Put a plan in place, and then do them. Have fun, challenge yourself and get yourself use to the feeling of being scared and stepping into the unknown.

Public speaking is one of the most frightening things for many other people to do and for me. So, to overcome my fear of public speaking, I joined Toast Masters. The first speech I gave was a nightmare. My knees were knocking (I didn't know that was possible – but it is!), and I broke out in a sweat, and my voice was a whisper when I started my speech.

I got through it, and though it wasn't the most remarkable speech, the exhilaration of actually overcoming my fear was terrific. After that, I kept going and now enjoy public speaking so much that I jump at any opportunity to speak.

5. Focus on Living a Balanced and Healthy Life

"To keep the body in good health is a duty…otherwise, we shall not be able to keep the mind strong and clear."

– Buddha

Version One is Better Than Version None

Living a balanced and healthy, active life builds our resilience and ability to successfully manage the disruption that change can have on our lives.

Stress is a normal response to dealing with changes and challenges in daily life. In the short term, stress can help you perform better under pressure, but constant stress can pose problems for your health.

Finding positive ways to deal with the stress and pressure that we face daily is key to our survival on both a physical and emotional level.

Some healthy lifestyle actions you can use to manage change and disruption in your life successfully are:

- Eat a healthy diet.

- Exercise regularly.

- Reduce caffeine and sugar.

- Avoid cigarettes, alcohol, and other drugs.

- Get enough sleep.

- Practice mediation regularly

- Take time out and disconnect from technology

- Learn how to relax and have fun

- Connect with others. Spend time with people who have a positive impact on your life.

There are many more things you can do to live a healthy balanced life. The key is that you commit to activities that enable you to be resilient, optimistic, physically and mentally fit to successful work through the impact of change on your life.

Key Take Away

1. Change your habits to change the life.

2. Emotional pain is momentary; the pain, later on, is reflection.

Chapter Twenty-One: Richness of Human Life

"Happiness is not by chance, but by choice."

-Jim Rohn

Have you anytime thought about why most of us find ourselves increasingly upset, depressed, helpless, anxious, or unhappy despite noticeable prosperity and sufficient resources available handy? Broadly speaking, nearly 95% of us are feeling that lack of manners or improper behavior in everyday social intercourse, even with nears and dears to getting worse. In addition, more than 80% feel rejected, demeaned, or humiliated even in the job environment, although the organizations are profit-making.

We have lost respect for each other and never realize till we have dire consequences later. With an incident in West Bengal before a decade, I was astonished when the will of a chartered accountant was declared to donate his whole property to his servant who was taking care of him day and night in his grey days. Because his wife and grown-up children ignored him, his family had taken it for granted that they would enjoy the inherited resources when the older man would leave for heavenly abode. But later on, they realized that they did not even have proper shelter for living.

In my banking career, I came across many cases when the head of the family opted for 'Former or survivor' instead of 'Either or survivor' for a mode of operation of fixed deposits. Because they thought if total money is transferred to their survivors, they may not treat him properly during the later part of his life.

Life Of Survival

When we check the history, we find that in olden days human was living with great difficulties. The human struggled to live in the caves by protecting himself from the external environment like attacks from wild animals, inadequate weather conditions, and feeding himself. He killed some animals and ate them for survival. More giant animals were killing smaller ones, and the fittest always survived.

In the existing environment, humans still have the same concept, "Fittest survives." A prominent businessman hunts the smaller one. One becomes rich by extracting money and resources from the other. Earlier stresses of humans were compensated by defending themselves against wild animals and environmental threats by running away and hiding at safe places. They had very few external attacks, and therefore they faced fewer stresses and survived. In today's environment, man has many external attacks like lack of money, proper shelter, improper jobs, taxations, political interferences, etc. And therefore, the amount of stress has increased due to various strains, weakening their health and fitness. A man in the job constantly fears threats to be fired and therefore saves his skin first and does not utilize his full potential to give desired profitability. But anyhow, he survives and lives and completes his life span despite specific difficulties.

A person survives despite complicated relationships, severe financial hardship, death of a loved one, serious health issues. They are just alive and stretch the surface of who they are beyond what they have endured. Their lives are built upon the pain of their past. Their identities are bound and tied up in what happened to them. They live with survival badges outside but living wounded from inside. His natural abilities, hidden talents, and desires remain dormant and never reach their full potential.

Life Of Success

The paradigm shifts from survival to success over time for some individuals according to their perception of success. Some of them take success as an act of revenge. For most of them, power, popularity, position, and better jobs are defined as success. Despite having branded clothes, imported cars, lovely houses, and shiny ornaments, they are miserable and hopeless. We have observed some celebrities living with subject lifestyles and materialistic wealth but commit suicide due to unresolved issues and lack of desired characteristic value.

Their outward appearance is like the teeth of an elephant; they have faulty inward perception. As a result, we have seen some high-profile sportsmen, athletes, business people even ministers with hidden issues and unresolved messes. Confidential matters are shocking when shameful and painful dealings are exposed; their so-called successful lives tremble negatively.

Life of Significance

A Life of Significance is a life of courage and bravery. It requires courage to unpack and unpeel the issues that keep us messy, out-of-balance or out-of-order. There is awareness among these people, and therefore they understand the higher level of living. They know that some of the pains in life are pains of change. Consequently, they accept and undergo required changes.

When you understand the value of pains and changes, you endure for some more time and bear the pain for longer. They agree with the quote of Napoleon that within every adversity is the seed to an equal or more significant benefit. They have deeply understood what Albert Einstein said that it's not that I'm so bright, it's just that I stay with problems longer.

Persons with a life of significance always rise above the survival and own success mentality. They are in a position to help others and live a life of joy for themselves and the happiness of others.

Intelligent Quotient

An intelligence quotient (IQ) is a total score derived from several standardized tests designed to assess human intelligence. The abbreviation "IQ" was coined by the psychologist William Stern for the German term Intelligenzquotient. His time for a scoring method for intelligence tests at the University of Breslau he advocated in a 1912 book.

Historically, IQ is a score obtained by dividing a person's mental age score, obtained by administering an intelligence test, by the person's chronological age, both expressed in years and months. The resulting fraction is multiplied by 100 to get the IQ score.

While IQ strives to measure some intelligence concepts, it may fail to measure broader definitions of intelligence accurately. IQ tests examine some areas of intelligence while neglecting others, such as creativity and social intelligence.

Emotional Quotient

An emotional quotient (EQ), also called an emotional intelligence quotient, is a measurement of a person's ability to monitor his or her emotions, cope with pressures and demands, and control his or her thoughts and actions. The ability to assess and affect situations and relationships with other people also plays a role in emotional intelligence. This measurement is intended to be a tool that is similar to the intelligence quotient (IQ), which is a measurement of a person's intellect. However, there is much debate surrounding the legitimacy of EQ, primarily because there is no standard of measurement.

Studies have been done on possible ways that a high or low EQ might affect a person's abilities to perform under pressure, resolve conflict, and cope with challenges. For example, someone who has a low EQ might lack self-confidence and be pessimistic, both of which might affect his or her performance when doing specific tasks. People who are not proponents of the concept believe that confidence, self-esteem, and attitude are simply personality matters, which cannot be measured or modified. Other studies have linked this measurement to communication skills and other social skills that people either lack or possess.

Spiritual Quotient

IQ looks at cognitive intelligence; EQ looks at the emotional power of a person. But the spiritual quotient (SQ) looks at the spiritual power of a person. Spirituality increases the ability of a person to be creative and to be aware and insightful. The concept of Spiritual Quotient (SQ) is fast emerging as the next significant aspect of scientific study as it directly correlates to a person's awareness and consciousness. Spirituality is the ability to recognize that there is intelligence beyond our five senses. There is a universal power that creates and governs everything within and beyond the worlds, we know, and that power is omnipresent. Spirituality exists within every individual. It is believed that whatever is available in-universe is also available within us.

Spiritual intelligence allows our inner values to drive through peaceful interactions with the world around us. It develops our concern for others, our respect for other living beings, and improves our conscious effort to make a positive contribution to society.

Key Take Away

1. "Spiritual intelligence is like a vaccination against greed, arrogance, and tyranny."-Saidi Mdala

2. "Spiritual Intelligence represents our drive for meaning and connection with the infinite."-Stephen Covey

Epilogue/Conclusion

The outlines discussed in the book have been chosen with an intention to cover the broader range from individual health and fitness to personal transformation for all age groups. In addition, examples and messages have been depicted in chapters to make the concept clearer. The references taken from the books and sites are the outcome of overall fruitful reading from books and various audios and podcasts.

In order to grow to the next version with gradual conditioning, a series of books have been generated. Still, intense learning from each chapter can more precisely be utilized if principles are applied deeply for the specific resolution of day-to-day life issues. Therefore, the book may work as a reference book rather than merely knowing the ways or tips. Most of the topics are based on psychology and natural linguistic exercises for specific issues.

I invite you to discuss any issues illustrated in the book or otherwise for mutual benefits. The contacts and site addresses are given at the end of this book.

Bibliography

1. ofpad.com

2. wanderlustworker.com

3. www.oprah.com

4. www.forbes.com

5. www.psychologytoday.com

6. www.forbes.com

Acknowledgments

I am thankful to my friends, family members, coworkers from public sector organizations, soldiers from Armed Forces, Government officials, author communities, and readers from aboard for their suggestions, feedback, and advice in writing and publishing the book.

About the Author

The author had 15 years of active service in Indian Air Force as an Airmen. He worked on Aero Engines of various aircraft equipped in the Armed forces. He was working in the trade of Engine fitter and had a specialization in Helicopter engines. During his service in Air Force, he was posted to different parts of the country, including Leh-Ladakh and Jammu, and Kashmir. He was part of the various operation of the Armed Forces like Blue start operation, Blast Track operation, and Passive air defense during peacetime. He worked in Air Force Units and rendered service in Army in units of Air Defence Regiments.

Along with the Equipment and Aircraft, he was also trained in Arms and ammunition like .303 rifles and LMGs. While working on the aircraft, he discharged the duties of Guard commander and preserved various security levels of Air Force at different units. As a senior noncommissioned officer, he also worked as a supervisor in canteen store departments and unit-run canteens. He recently published his military biography. Apart from the real-life story, the book '**What I will be remembered for**' also narrated the glimpses of various operations during wartime and familiarized various gallantry awards.

The author has published the self-help book '**Build Better Version Of Yourself**' with 21 psychological ways to organize the mind to help and make changes to eradicate and resolve significant issues faced by individuals. After it was widely accepted globally, another book in the series '**Explore Your Ideal Version**" was published to rediscover 21 Resilient Potentials Within individual.

The author was also a manager in the State Bank of India for 24 years in the supervisory cadre. He discharged the duties of a field officer, account officer, and branch manager in various branches of Gujarat. He had maintained and upgraded different departments as 'Exceptionally well run' and met the requirements of levels aspired by the Bank. During various line segment assignments, he managed men and material with adequate moral boosting of workers. He worked as a joint custodian of the Reserve Bank of India for several years. He maintained cash flow for ATM replenishments and Currency Administrative Cells of branches of SBI and other banks. He was also awarded as the best branch manager of State Bank of India in 2014-15.

The author had a master's in psychology in 1986 from one of the universities in South India. During his active service in the Armed forces and corporate sector, he guided organizations and individuals under his experiments and experiences to resolve day-to-day issues. He acquired computer skills by studying DISM and PGDCA from Saurashtra University and the degree from APTECH. While serving in the bank, he also imparted skills to students in his spare time with morning and evening classes by teaching them MS Office, C++, Visual FoxPro, visual basics, and website designing.

The author has a vocal and instrument playing hobby like harmonium, guitar, flute, mouth organ, and violin. Being an artist of All India Radio, he performed several programs over radio and stages in different parts of Gujarat. The author is presently working on varieties of niches in the form of books and videos on banking, meditation, motivation, music, and varied topics on personality traits and attitudinal effects on behavior exploring human psychology.

Author contacts:
krgoswami@krgoswami.com

krgoswami@live.com

krgoswami@gmail.com

Website:
https://krgoswami.com

Blog:
http://blog.krgoswami.com

http://academy.krgoswami.com

https://digitaleagleacademy.teachable.com